TREATMENT OF ADULT SURVIVORS OF INCEST

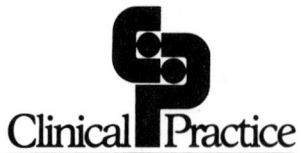

Clinical Practice

Number 27
Judith H. Gold, M.D., F.R.C.P.C.
Series Editor

TREATMENT OF ADULT SURVIVORS OF INCEST

Edited by

Patricia L. Paddison, M.D.

Psychiatrist, Center for Women's Health
The Virginia Mason Medical Center
Seattle, Washington

American
Psychiatric
Press, Inc.

Washington, DC
London, England

Copyright © 1993 American Psychiatric Press, Inc.
ALL RIGHTS RESERVED
Manufactured in the United States of America on acid-free paper
First Edition
96 95 94 93   4 3 2 1

American Psychiatric Press, Inc.
1400 K Street, N.W., Washington, DC 20005

Library of Congress Cataloging-in-Publication Data
Treatment of adult survivors of incest / edited by Patricia L.
    Paddison. — 1st ed.
        p.   cm. — (Clinical practice series: no. 27)
        Includes bibliographical references and index.
        ISBN 0-88048-469-1
        1. Incest victims—Rehabilitation—Congresses. 2. Psycho-
            therapy—
            Congresses. I. Paddison, Patricia L., 1951–   . II. Series.
        [DNLM: 1. Child Abuse, Sexual—therapy. 2. Child of Im-
            paired
    Parents—psychology. 3. Incest—psychology. 4. Psychotherapy—
    methods.   W1 CL767J no.27 / WM 610 T7834]
    RC560.I53T725 1993
    616.85′8369—dc20
    DNLM/DLC
    for Library of Congress   92-17653
                                                              CIP

British Library Cataloguing in Publication Data
A CIP record is available from the British Library.

Contents

Contributors

Jennifer D. Bolen, M.D.
Clinical Faculty, Department of Psychiatry, University
of Washington School of Medicine, Seattle, Washington

J. Case, M.D.
Psychiatric Director, Lipton II Women's Unit,
Charles River Hospital, Wellesley, Massachusetts

Robin G. Einbinder, C.S.W., M.P.H.
Associate Director, Rape Crisis Intervention Program,
Mount Sinai Medical Center, New York, New York

Denise J. Gelinas, Ph.D.
Private Practice, Northampton, Massachusetts;
Associate Professional Staff, Department of Psychiatry,
Bay State Medical Center, Springfield, Massachusetts

Jean M. Goodwin, M.D., M.P.H.
Professor, Psychiatry and Behavioral Sciences,
University of Texas Medical Branch, Galveston, Texas

Richard J. Loewenstein, M.D.
Senior Psychiatrist, Director, Dissociative Disorders Program,
Sheppard and Enoch Pratt Hospital, Baltimore, Maryland; Assistant
Clinical Professor, Department of Psychiatry
and Behavioral Medicine, University of Maryland
School of Medicine, Baltimore, Maryland

Ellen Maker, B.S.
Medical Student, Mount Sinai Medical Center,
New York, New York

Patricia L. Paddison, M.D.
Psychiatrist, Center for Women's Health,
The Virginia Mason Medical Center, Seattle, Washington

José A. Saporta, Jr., M.D.
Staff Psychiatrist, Charles River Hospital; Clinical Associate
in Psychiatry, Massachusetts General Hospital; Instructor
in Psychiatry, Harvard Medical School, Boston, Massachusetts

James J. Strain, M.D.
Director, Behavioral Medicine and Consultation Division
of Psychiatry, and Professor of Psychiatry,
Mount Sinai Medical Center, New York, New York

Introduction
to the Clinical Practice Series

*O*ver the years of its existence the series of monographs entitled *Clinical Insights* gradually became focused on providing current, factual, and theoretical material of interest to the clinician working outside of a hospital setting. To reflect this orientation, the name of the Series has been changed to *Clinical Practice.*

The Clinical Practice Series will provide books that give the mental health clinician a practical, clinical approach to a variety of psychiatric problems. These books will provide up-to-date literature reviews and emphasize the most recent treatment methods. Thus, the publications in the Series will interest clinicians working both in psychiatry and in the other mental health professions.

Each year a number of books will be published dealing with all aspects of clinical practice. In addition, from time to time when appropriate, the publications may be revised and updated. Thus, the Series will provide quick access to relevant and important areas of psychiatric practice. Some books in the Series will be authored by a person considered to be an expert in that particular area; others will be edited by such an expert, who will also draw together other knowledgeable authors to produce a comprehensive overview of that topic.

Some of the books in the Clinical Practice Series will have their foundation in presentations at an annual meeting of the American Psychiatric Association. All will contain the most recently available information on the subjects discussed. Theoretical and scientific data will be applied to clinical situations, and case illustrations will be utilized in order to make the material even more relevant for the practitioner. Thus, the Clinical Practice Series should provide educational reading in a compact format especially designed for the mental health clinician–psychiatrist.

Judith H. Gold, M.D., F.R.C.P.C.
Series Editor
Clinical Practice Series

Clinical Practice Series Titles

Preface

*I*n the fall of 1986, I began my fellowship and began seeing patients in a Premenstrual Syndromes (PMS) Clinic at Mount Sinai Medical Center in New York City. As part of the routine screening, I asked about adverse sexual experiences about 30 minutes into the interview. Specifically, I asked, "Has anyone ever touched you against your will in childhood or adulthood?" About 9 months into the fellowship, I began to wonder if there was an epidemic of childhood sexual abuse or if this was somehow linked to PMS. I had never received any education about sexual abuse in my residency and yet so many PMS patients (many who had been in therapy) said, "I've never told this to anyone before." I ultimately published a paper on PMS and sexual abuse and began working as a Psychiatric Consultant to the Mount Sinai Hospital Rape Crisis Intervention Program (Paddison et al. 1990). Robin Einbinder, C.S.W., M.P.H., and I devised a standardized intake interview for group treatment of incest survivors and decided to try to document group outcome.

In the process of running incest survivors' groups, I attended a comprehensive course in May 1990 called "Psychological Trauma," sponsored by the Harvard Medical School Department of Continuing Education and the Massachusetts Mental Health Center Department of Psychiatry and Trauma Clinic. The course directors were Bessel van der Kolk, M.D., and Lawrence Lifson, M.D. This course was finally the "sit-down dinner" I needed for clinically comprehensive and relevant treatment of survivors of incest instead of the "appetizers" I had been experiencing. Judith Herman, M.D., received a standing ovation at this conference and deserved it for being willing to pioneer this work when it was still being silenced in our profession. To sit in a room filled with over 300 clinicians, all doing group therapy with survivors, discussing the pros and cons of various approaches to incest groups, inspired me to try to get together a group of clinicians to present a symposium at the American Psychiatric Association that would be relevant to other psychiatrists and would outline different modalities for treatment.

This book is an expansion of a symposium presented at the 144th

Annual Meeting of the American Psychiatric Association in New Orleans, Louisiana, in May 1991. Unfortunately, Judith Herman, M.D., our original discussant, had prior writing commitments and could not write our discussion, but Jean M. Goodwin, M.D., M.P.H., another pioneer in the field of incest survivors, has honored the book by taking on the task of synthesizing this material and commenting on the Seduction Hypothesis in Chapter 6, "The Seduction Hypothesis 100 Years After."

Chapter 1, "Relational Patterns in Incestuous Families, Malevolent Variations, and Specific Interventions With the Adult Survivor" by Denise Gelinas, Ph.D., examines the relational issues that abound in individual as well as group treatment of incest survivors. Understanding and appreciating the tenacity of family connections is an essential aspect of any treatment, especially with incest survivors, for whom family issues usually complicate the treatment process. Chapter 2, "Group Treatment With Incest Survivors," presents an overview of group treatment as well as the results of a group outcome study I completed at the Mount Sinai Medical Center Rape Crisis Intervention Program, along with my colleagues Robin G. Einbinder, C.S.W., M.P.H., Ellen Maker, B.S., and James J. Strain, M.D. It also contains a brief review of the prevalence data of sexual abuse.

"Sexuality-Focused Treatment With Survivors and Their Partners" (Chapter 3) by Jennifer D. Bolen, M.D., is an important guiding light to clinicians, because so little is published in this area and yet as many as 80% of incest survivors in my group treatment study reported sexual dysfunction.

Richard J. Loewenstein, M.D., explores the vast realm of dissociation in its complex clinical presentation and also presents practical approaches to its symptom formation in Chapter 4, "Aspects of the Treatment of Dissociative Disorders in Survivors of Incest." Chapter 5, "The Role of Medications in Treating Adult Survivors of Childhood Trauma" by José A. Saporta, Jr., M.D., and J. Case, M.D., offers a systematic format, based on the psychobiology of trauma, to clinicians wondering when to intervene with medications, what to use, and for what duration of treatment.

This book attempts to broaden the clinician's treatment options and to provide education on the multidimensional approach to the treatment of incest survivors that is necessary to facilitate healing. Individual therapy is an important mainstay, and the additional modalities presented here will in no way replace or diminish its importance. It was beyond the scope of this book to adequately cover the issues of individual therapy with incest survivors, but I will issue a warning about remaining "morally neutral" with these patients: this neutrality may be experienced as judging, maintaining the secrecy, or siding with the perpetrator. These patients need to hear the words "it wasn't your fault, he [or she] was wrong to have done it." And of course, many survivors will continue to blame themselves or feel responsible despite hearing to the contrary.

I would like to acknowledge and thank the survivors who agreed to participate and to share their experiences in group treatment. This book would probably not have been conceived without their participation, because the original idea for the symposium centered around presenting my group work. The group therapy with incest survivors has been some of the most emotionally demanding work I have ever done, but also the most rewarding. The strength of these women in their struggles with recovery has touched me deeply.

I would also like to thank all survivors and treating clinicians for helping to remove the shroud of secrecy surrounding incest. The improvement of treatment cannot occur without survivors' participation and feedback. We must be willing to examine failed as well as successful treatment to understand how to further healing. Most importantly, issues surrounding the *prevention* of childhood abuse have not been adequately addressed or funded. Why is this epidemic occurring? What can be done to stop it?

A special note of acknowledgment is also due to the Rape Crisis Intervention Program at the Mount Sinai Medical Center for the support of this work—in particular, Iona Siegel, M.S.W., director; Robin Einbinder, C.S.W., M.P.H., assistant director; Kathy Teets-Grimm, M.D., medical director; and Angela Diaz, M.D., director of the Adolescent Health Center at Mount Sinai, who gave much needed support and feedback. My thanks to Ellen Maker, B.S., medical student, for helping with many aspects of our study. I also owe many thanks to Jim Strain, M.D., not only for his assistance on this project, but also for being a very nurturing mentor who has helped my education and promoted my career and personal development.

A special note of thanks to Jennifer D. Bolen, M.D., Director of the Center for Women's Health at the Virginia Mason Medical Center, for being a colleague and a friend who creates a sympathetic and supportive work environment in which to continue my work with survivors. I would also like to acknowledge the efforts and support of another colleague, Marcia Robbins, M.S.W., who helped Dr. Bolen and me with editing and suggestions and who is a valued member of our division. Finally, my thanks to Jane Lopez, who was helpful to both Dr. Bolen and me with the editing of our chapters.

Patricia L. Paddison, M.D.

Reference

Paddison PL, Gise LH, Lebovits A: Sexual abuse and premenstrual syndrome: comparison between a lower and higher socioeconomic group. Psychosomatics 31:265–272, 1990

Relational Patterns in Incestuous Families, Malevolent Variations, and Specific Interventions With the Adult Survivor

Denise J. Gelinas, Ph.D.

Relationally Based Abuse and Amplification of the Trauma Response

Incestuous abuse constitutes a particular type of trauma. The fact that it occurs *within* the family introduces issues of "agency" and "relationship" into the abuse, which amplify the trauma responses of the child. When treating the adult incest survivor, it is important to understand and address these relationally based aspects of incest, or full therapeutic resolution of the trauma is precluded. The relational elements are an intrinsic part of the trauma itself, not extraneous complications, and they should be explicitly and directly addressed in the therapy of the adult incest survivor.

In this chapter, I will examine how incestuous agency and relationship are experienced by the child and how these relational structures amplify the child's trauma response. The focus will then shift from the child's experience of the family structures to a clinical description of the most usual relational patterns found in incestuous families.

One important relational variant will be introduced—incest with "malevolent intent." Incest with malevolent intent is particularly destructive in its effects on both the family structure and the child's phenomenology; the concept can serve as a bridge between the child's phenomenology and the structure of many incestuous families. Unfortunately, it is not uncommon. The term "malevolent intent" is being introduced in the hopes that description and labelling will help clinicians recognize when they are treating its effects. For most clinicians, encounters with the effects of real malevolence can be intellectually confusing and emotionally taxing. Having a working description can help with recognition, intervention, and countertransference. Finally, some specific interventions for treating the relational issues of incest will be described. The early relational patterns of the family characteristically recur in the adolescent and adult life of the survivor. These patterns can be tenacious and need to be addressed in therapy. Some approaches have proved helpful, and these will be described in detail.

Agency Versus Facticity

In clinical work with incest survivors, it is helpful to remember that incest is a trauma of agency rather than of facticity (Gelinas 1990). Facticity can be thought of as the objective, factual bases of reality in a person's life that occur and have occurred through happenstance, accident, unintentional event, or simple luck. Facticity might include gender at birth, genetic material, physical health, nationality and/or racial grouping at birth, and occurrences and events of development such as hereditary diseases or parental divorce. None of these elements is planned, yet all have significant influence on a person's life (Boszormenyi-Nagy and Krasner 1986).

When someone falls and breaks a leg, that is facticity; if someone intentionally breaks another person's leg, that is agency. Accidents partake of facticity. But when somebody *does* something, that is usually agency. Intent and action by another person characterize agency. When considering something like trauma, facticity versus agency can make a great deal of difference. It is one thing to have a leg broken, or an eye put out in an auto accident; it is a very different thing to have someone intentionally break one's leg or put out one's eye. That injury didn't just happen, it was done.

In such a circumstance, the meaning of the event is changed, as is the intensity of the victim's response. When an injury or injustice is done, it hurts worse. Incest is a trauma of agency. Someone is doing something to a child, and that makes it worse for the child than if he or she were injured accidentally. Even young children can differentiate agency from facticity, and we can hear it in their statements at play. One child might say to another, "But it was an accident," in an attempt to change the meaning of an injury or unfairness, and perhaps to avoid blame. A typical rejoinder might be, "Uh-uh, you did it on purpose!" and the battle is joined. Or an adult may attempt to explain to a child that a favorite toy was not broken or ruined by another child, but by the rain, or the wind, or the simple passage of time. If the child can understand this, it makes a difference, and the experience of injury is not as bad.

Actually, agency makes a difference for all of us. For example, there was a medium-size tree outside the building where my office is. I find that it bothers me that inexplicably, someone vandalized that tree and killed it. It would be different if the tree had been knocked over by hurricane winds that had hit New England. That would have been sad; the fact that someone had such an intent, and took the time and trouble to kill the tree, leaves me with a more complicated emotional response. Agency always complicates matters.

Trauma in Relationship

Incest is also a "relationally based" form of chronic abuse and trauma. Like spouse-battering or the physical abuse of a child, it occurs within the family unit, at the hands of people with whom the victim is in relation. This implies that the child's relational life will be distorted in adolescence and adulthood as a result of the very significant distortions in her* early relational life. The therapist will encounter these distortions in both the survivor's current relationships and in the therapeutic relationship.

It is also important to recognize that when trauma occurs *within* a relationship, the extent and intensity of the "traumatic response" itself is amplified. For some reason, the mental health field has been somewhat slow to appreciate this fact, although other groups have not. For example, the practitioners of political torture have long been aware of this, and they use relationship in the service of their own aims. One way they do this is to use an ongoing relationship with one specific torturer,

---

*The feminine pronoun will be used for the incest survivor and the masculine for the offender. This reflects the predominant gender ratios in incest, but I want to draw attention to the fact that there are substantial numbers of male incest survivors and female incest offenders. My use of language is meant to simplify presentation, not to eliminate these other groups from consideration.

who combines authority and total control with physical torture and pretends the abuse is happening *because* of the prisoner's behavior. This is clearly nonsense; the prisoner is completely helpless, and a great deal of political torture is used to terrorize populations and not to gain information. The parallels with a child in a severely abusive family are quite clear, with the added unfortunate angle that this is occurring in the child's developmental context, so that besides heightened trauma, there are character developmental implications (Gelinas 1983).

Another illustrative example from torture's corrupted use of relationship to heighten trauma is the use of two-person teams, in which one individual is tough and the other solicitous. This technique uses the continuing relationship with the prisoner to exploit the vulnerability and trust elicited in the presence of the ostensibly more solicitous torturer. More subtly, this relational technique confuses the context; after all, does it really make sense for the prisoner to trust either one of these people? But the intense emotional field of the relational situation makes it unlikely that the prisoner will be able to remember that neither should be trusted—and very difficult to not feel grateful to the solicitous torturer. For a child being abused within the family, the potential for confusion and unwarranted trust and dependence is of course even greater. Especially when the incestuous parent is both abusive and then solicitous, it is impossible for the child to accurately understand what is going on or to remember to remain emotionally neutral and disengaged.

It is somewhat silly to think that a child *could* remain emotionally disengaged. As Winnicott pointed out, relational dependency is the central element in human development (Phillips 1988). It is needed for development, and the fact that the child was born into an abusive family does not change the child's need for relationship and dependency to be able to develop.

Herman (1990) pointed out that the symptoms shown by adults after political torture are nearly identical to the symptoms shown by battered women and by incest survivors. Goodwin (1991) has noted that the abusive and coercive techniques used in incest are many of the same ones used in political torture, by criminal sadists, in pornography, and in certain cult and religious practices. In all of these practices, relationship is used to heighten certain effects, often the degree of trauma experienced by the victim. When this combination is directed onto a child, the effects are both traumatic and developmental.

There are a number of reasons why the relational basis of incest amplifies the trauma response compared to nonrelational sexual abuse. The relational aspect of the abuse can specifically affect the child's perceptions of reality, emotions, and sense of self.

Perceptions and Reality

The child's phenomenology. In the case of incest, the abusing parent is not abusing the child 24 hours a day. During the day, or when around other people, the abuser is what could be called a regular person. But the person the child knows during the day or when around other people usually seems quite different to the child from the person when he or she is abusing that child. Incest survivors describe, in considerable frightened detail, how different that person seemed—in size and appearance, demeanor, expression, and even smell. Particularly when the abuse occurs only at night, then that nighttime abuser is very different than the parent or relative the child has known.

Patients frequently relate that the abuser would begin the abuse while they were asleep and would not speak while abusing them; this of course would heighten that sense of the parent changing. When the parent becomes that nighttime abuser, he or she "turns"—that is, becomes someone or something different from who the child has known for so long.

The turning described by many patients leads one to wonder whether this kind of transformation, especially in a parent, is an origin of the transcultural stories of individuals turning into creatures profoundly other than the familiar, known person. The Jekyll-and-Hyde transformation and the legends of the vampire and the werewolf come to mind here. The "other" seems always to be evil, frightening, inhumanly strong and powerful, and often perversely sexual. These are precisely the changes patients note when describing changing or turning of the parent during the actual episodes of abuse. The extent and thoroughness of such changes would of course be magnified if an abusing parent were significantly dissociated, or worse, had multiple personality disorder (MPD).

It is much more frightening to have a parent turn and do something traumatic than have that same activity occur at the hands of a stranger. That turning in itself is frightening. Where has the parent gone, and who or what is this? Will the real parent return? Has this one hurt or killed the real parent?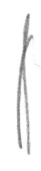

When a parent turns, the child becomes confused and frightened. The familiar has become strange, and that sort of thing is deeply unsettling. (It is one thing to be confronted with something new or strange; it is very different to have something one thought one knew *become* strange.)

For any of us, this kind of transformation could lead us to mistrust our own perceptions and interpretations or to question the nature of reality; for a child, with much less experience in the world, it is even more confusing. She may tacitly question her own abilities to perceive and make sense of people and the world. An incest survivor alludes to that in *Growing Through the Pain* (1989), when she titles one of her chapters "Specific Effects of Incest Trauma: 'Am I Crazy or Does Everybody See Lizards Dining Out in Washington, D.C.?'" What the child had known about *who* that parent was has needed dreadful revision. Alternatively, this could lead a child to the conclusion that her perceptions had been okay; it was simply that *the person* was not (i.e., that reality was tricky or changed). Unfortunately for the child, the focus of this revision is not a peripheral element in her life (such as a summer camp counselor, a movie, or some such thing) but is one of the most central aspects of her life and development.

With repetitions (of these changes or turnings in the nature of reality), the child begins to occupy a highly precarious place in relation to reality, never being really sure what is real and whether or how long it will remain so. She may come to believe that reality may be real, for now, but that in no way implies that what is reality now will be real in a couple of hours. That may connote to her that everything is real but changes, or that what appears to be reality is merely an evanescent surface, with a depth that is different showing itself only occasionally; worse, reality may have no depth. All of these tacit confusions may be associated with feelings of dread. These kind of questions have occupied the philosophically inclined for some time, but these individuals have usually been adult, have had the benefits of childhood, and to some extent could walk away from these questions when they so choose. Obviously, a 5-, or 7-, or 9-year-old cannot. She can never gain a trusting foothold about the nature of reality and her own relationship to it.

Ironically, the abuse to which she is being subjected is one of the most real things she experiences (in part because of the intense physicality of the experiences), but in many ways, this too can seem quite unbelievable. She may wonder who would believe that this is happening. For that matter, she may well not really know what this is. Also, these experiences would be affected by significant amounts of dissociation, which can make reality testing even more difficult. Finally, whatever efforts the abuser made at mystification would further confuse the child. These processes, in turn, cause the child to further doubt her own capabilities in knowing what she knows; she has neither an exterior frame of reference nor a verbal analysis for what is happening. All of these processes actively contribute to her confusion, fear, and experience of being thoroughly overwhelmed, and thus amplify the extent to which she has been traumatized.

These are some of the reasons why, in therapy, the adult incest survivor may return again and again to the question of whether all these things that she can remember really happened. These processes can also help therapists understand why incest survivors could find themselves persuaded by disbelieving therapists that these events had not taken place. Of course, the symptoms and lasting negative effects did not resolve in the context of such poor treatment. But the tampering with reality that occurs with incest can help clinicians understand how incest survivors could be authoritatively persuaded against knowing what they knew.

Dissociation.   Moving the perspective now from the child's phenomenology to Pierre Janet's terms, the child cannot explain, or fit, her experiences within her current cognitive schema. As Janet (1889/1973) put it:

> Under ordinary circumstances, people automatically integrate new information, by taking appropriate action without paying much conscious attention to what is happening. . . . The memory system maintains coherence of mental functioning and links the present with the past by continually organizing and categorizing new information. (Translated and quoted in van der Kolk and van der Hart 1989, p. 1531)

Janet (1889/1973) also thought that integration into memory depended on the cognitive assessment of all new experiences, and that experiences that were quite frightening or novel might not fit into a person's existing cognitive schema (van der Kolk and van der Hart 1989, p. 1532).

For the incestuously abused child, the magnitude of the novel stimulation, the physical and emotional responses, and the parental turning make this cognitive work impossible. The experiences are too much and too strange to integrate. Sexual abuse by a stranger would be difficult to make sense of because of the physical sensation and the child's physical responses. Incestuous abuse is complicated by the novel experiences of parental turning and the child's complicated emotional responses. As a result, the child's cognitive appraisal of the situation is severely impaired. This forces this material to remain unintegrated and sometimes unremembered.

Emotions and Affect

If this material is then linked with what Janet (1909) referred to as vehement emotion, the trauma response is further exacerbated. The occurrence of trauma within the relational context can be counted on to exacerbate the affective response of the child. There is an emotional attachment between parent and child, or at the very least, the need for attachment by the child. Whenever a parent and child interact, their activity is embedded in an emotional context based on their relational history. The child's trust, love, dependence, reliance, and predisposition to be soothed and comforted are called up when in contact with the parent. One of the primary developmental functions a parent serves is to help the child regulate his or her level of stimulation. When a parent or other relationally intimate person abuses a child, the abuse, like all activity, occurs in the presence of the emotional context of the relationship.

The emotional attachments to that parent have been elicited by the presence of the parent *and become involved in the child's response to the trauma.* When a parent turns, the emotions that the child feels about that parent increase the alarm and fear the child experiences. In other words, the presence of the preexisting feelings potentiate the feelings prompted by the abuse.

Dissociation.   Again, moving from the child's phenomenology to an explanatory framework, Janet's work is helpful. When "trying to account for what interferes with the integration of experience," Janet (1909) wrote, "I was led to recognize in many subjects the role of one or several events in their past life. These events, which were accompanied by a vehement emotion and a destruction of the psychological system, had left traces"(translated and quoted in van der Kolk and van der Hart 1989, p. 1532).

Unfortunately for incestuously abused children, the intensity of the vehement emotion, which (in Janet's thinking) determines the lasting impact of the trauma, depends on both the emotional state of the victim at the time of the event and on the cognitive appraisal of the experiences. I have already noted here that certain relational issues (turning and the child's complicated emotional response to the *parent's* doing these things) complicate the cognitive appraisal of the incestuous abuse. At this point, the issue of vehement emotion arises. Because the mere presence of the parent usually elicits emotions in a child, and the presence of these emotions potentiates those experienced when the parent abuses the child, the vehement emotion experienced by the child is severe.

Thus, both the cognitive appraisal and the emotional intensity of the trauma are complicated by the relational base of the trauma. These need to be kept in mind by the therapist, regardless of the age of the survivor or the time elapsed since the abuse ended.

The child's phenomenology.   When a parent sexually abuses a child in the context of these emotions, these preexisting emotions themselves also become contaminated. Usually the child's feelings of security and safety oscillate hopefully for a time with feelings of fear and disbelief. But with repeated turnings and trauma, security and safety become the hypervigilant scanning of the parent and the environment. Trust is seriously compromised, and this distrust generalizes to all relationships, expressing itself finally in the therapy as wariness and continual testing. Dependency becomes a baffled depression, and joy seems to wither and become foreign to the child.

Most importantly, the child finds that she is being abused *within* what had been her safe base, and so she no longer has a safe base in the world. This increases her experience of isolation and hypervigilance, taints her perception of the world, and teaches her that she must cope as best she can alone, because there appears to be no one in the world to whom she can turn. Obviously, this affects her later coping skills, particularly because all this learning has been tacit and she has no verbal analysis of it.

If, however, the child has a nurturant relationship with some adult outside the abusing family, this protects her to some extent. The presence of a nurturant grandparent, mother of a friend, or mentor can mitigate some of the confusion, fear and isolation of incestuous abuse, even if that adult does not know of the abuse. The very fact of that nurturing relationship and the experiences the child has within that relationship can be saving.

Sense of Self

The child's sense of self also takes a battering during incestuous abuse. The relationship with a parent can be a powerful stabilizing and comforting force for a child in coping with an external threat. But when a parent incestuously abuses a child, that threat can no longer be said to be entirely external. For the child—who is still actively forming relational templates and internalizing her parents and others around her—when one of the parents abuses, it is not clear to the child that this abuser is entirely on the outside. Some of that abuser is already in her head and heart. And so, who is abusing? (Her ego boundaries are not yet firm, and trauma overwhelms ego boundaries anyway. That is one of the definitions of trauma.)

We see the effects of this particular process most vividly when we encounter persecutory alters in patients with MPD. These persecutory alters usually started as protective, but in the face of their own helplessness to stop the abuse, they gradually became persecutory. This, it seems to me, is an internalization of a developmental part of the child that expresses the changing experience of the child and also of the offender! The offender's experience of self has often undergone the shift from protective to persecutory with respect to the child he or she is abusing.

A related set of concerns is: can the abused child really afford to see the incest as abuse? Is *it* bad, or is it she herself who is bad? These concerns seem to me to be some of the origins of the vertical splitting that Shengold (1979, 1989) described so vividly and Summit extended and embedded in his classic work on the Child Sexual Abuse Accommodation Syndrome (1983).

Shengold (1989) described this combination of denial, distortion, compartmentalization, and confusion as resulting specifically from parental abuse, and noted the importance of the relational base for the vertical splitting:

> If the child must turn to the very parent who inflicts abuse and who is felt as bad for relief of the distress that the parent has caused, then the child must break with what has been experienced and out of a desperate need for rescue, must register the parent, *delusionally,* [Shengold's emphasis] as good. Only the mental image of a good parent who will rescue can help the child deal with the terrifying intensity of fear and rage that is the effect of the tormenting experiences. The alternative—to maintain the overwhelming stimulation and bad parental image—means annihilation of identity, the feeling of the self. So the bad has to be registered as good. This is a mind-splitting or mind-fragmenting operation. To survive, such children must keep in some compartment of their minds, the delusion of good parents and the delusive promise that all the terror, pain, and rage will be transformed into love. These need not be psychotic delusions—neurotic delusions are frequent enough. . . . The child's mind is split into contradictory fragments to separate the bad from the good (Ferenczi 1933/1955). I am describing not schizophrenia . . . but the establishment of isolated divisions of the mind in which contradictory images of the self and of the parents are never permitted to coalesce. This compartmentalized "vertical splitting" transcends diagnostic categories. Feeling and thinking are compromised; registration of what has happened and what is happening is divided into "compartments" and therefore is inadequate. (pp. 26–27)

And so, the development of the sense of self is profoundly compromised, as are the relational templates the child will be relying on for the rest of her life and the development of clear and robust feelings and thinking.

When a child is incestuously abused, she is being chronically traumatized *within* her own developmental context, which pervasively contaminates that child's developmental context, *by* someone of that family (often the child's parent). The child is thus tacitly faced with attempting to grow and develop in a severely distorted developmental context, with access only to distorted relationships. The character implications have been delineated.

The characteristic negative effects of incest were initially noted to be posttraumatic stress syndromes (PTSD), with secondary elaborations arising from lack of appropriate treatment, continuing relational imbalances, and intergenerational risk of incest (Gelinas 1983). Many clinicians found the PTSD notion persuasive and helpful, but were less able, cognitively and emotionally, to attend to the relational aspects of the model. Perhaps relational problems and effects are not as succinctly described, and they certainly have little space in DSM-III-R (American Psychiatric Association 1987) nomenclature, which aspires to different purposes. But noting the combined relational and traumatic aspects of incest is essential to providing good treatment of its effects.

These combined relational and traumatic aspects differentiate incest from other forms of trauma and continue in the survivor's life long after the sexually abusive episodes have stopped. The relationally based aspects of the trauma contribute to the particular trauma responses the survivor experiences, the construction of the survivor's self, and the development of the survivor's character structure and object relations. Ironically, the families that can produce such pervasive distortions in development may look, superficially, quite normal and functional.

Characteristic Relational Patterns in Incestuous Families

Incestuous abuse usually develops over time—the result of individual, dyadic, systemic, and role-related patterns that converge and devalue at least one child and (because of tacit personal and family decisions) may increase the probability of incest or decrease it.

The development of the incestuous abuse is intimately linked to family functioning in several ways. The abuser has responsibility for the onset and continuation of the abuse, but the family functioning contributes to the likelihood of its beginning and continuing. It should be noted here that examining the involvement of the family system is in no way an argument for blaming the family for the onset of incest, nor is it an attempt to remove responsibility for the abuse from the adult abuser. The person who perpetrates the abuse bears the responsibility (Gelinas 1983, 1986, 1988). But it is helpful, therapeutically and preventively, to know that certain patterns are frequently associated with incest. Some families can be thought of as being on the fast track for incest: they are making tacit decisions and leading their lives in ways that progressively increase the probability that incest will occur. On the other hand, families can make decisions and function in ways that progressively decrease the probability of incest. The family's development can resemble a stochastic process, where decisions increasingly shunt them in one direction or another.

Parentification

The process of parentification is usually important in the development of incest. (The material in this section is summarized and extended from earlier work [Gelinas 1983].) Parentification describes the processes by which a child takes on duties that are greater than those that would be age-appropriate. As Boszormenyi-Nagy and Spark (1984) and Boszormenyi-Nagy and Krasner (1986) have pointed out:

> As a transactional shift of role boundaries, parentification is not necessarily detrimental to a child. In fact, it can be a child's appropriate adaptation to temporary family strain. In these situations, a youngster can benefit from learning about responsible role taking. From a contextual perspective, parentification is destructive when it depletes a child's resources and trust reserves. This occurs when adults manipulate their offspring's innate tendency for trusting devotion. (1986, p. 419)

In families where there is incest, parentification of one devalued child is a pervasive and permanent developmental stance. Intrinsic to this process within these families are the transfer of task functions and responsibility and the lack of fairness between obligations and entitlements.

In parentification, a child performs task functions that are excessive and premature for her age and developmental level. Through usually unwitting induction by the parents, she also begins to assume *responsibility* for these functions. She may become prematurely responsible for the cleaning, cooking, shopping, yardwork, billpaying, and/or child care. She may, for instance, increasingly be called upon to take care of her younger sibs, but not for discrete periods of time, nor in a paid capacity, nor in any format that recognizes this as an important and valued function. Instead, the child care tasks are excessive, yet increasingly her responsibility. It is not uncommon to find that a 9-year-old girl has been handed an infant in the family to care for. It may become the parentified child's responsibility to remember to come home directly after school to take care of her sibs, to remember the children's lessons and doctor's appointments and take them there, to see that they are dressed appropriately, and to remain home from school with them when they are sick. (We see here the processes described by Herman [1981] whereby the incest victim is increasingly isolated within her own family, from her siblings and her mother.) In the family's thinking, the parents should not miss work or other activities, but it gradually no longer occurs to anyone that the parentified child should not miss school! Her legitimate needs and rights are gradually eclipsed.

One 12-year-old child I treated appeared for her first meeting wearing an old-fashioned housedress. She had been sexually abused by her father for 6 years and had disclosed this to a school counselor, who made the appointment for her. The girl's parents knew nothing about the appointment, and she appeared surprised that this was unusual. She was very parentified—tightly controlled and businesslike. Toward the end of the meeting, I said that we needed to make arrangements to have her family come in too and that I would call them to schedule their appointments. She told me not to bother, that she took care of the scheduling—whereupon she removed a datebook (with pink bunnies on the cover) and proceeded to talk with me about scheduling. I acquiesced in this enterprise for this session but asked her about the papers hanging out of her datebook. Matter-of-factly, she showed me that they were an array of bills. She had put each in the book exactly 1 week before it was due, at which point she would inform the parents that she needed a check for a certain amount payable to whomever had issued the bill. As it turned out, the girl was also responsible for reminding her mother to be sure to put in her dentures before going to work! This 12-year-old child dressed decades older than her age and functioned as a well-organized 30-year-old, but at significant cost to her development. We had a good idea where to start with this family before we had even done the full family evaluation.

Over time, the parentified child begins to meet the needs of the family to the exclusion of her own, as she has gradually adopted the role of a parent, which is nearly unilateral when caring for infants and young children. That is, a parent has nearly unilateral obligations to care for a young child, but the young child has no *obligation* to care for the parent in return. The child may develop loyalty, but that is not the same as obligation. A parentified child is taught to put everyone's needs before her own, but she has had to do this while still a child, without having had the opportunity to complete many of the developmental tasks of childhood. In time, she may no longer realize that she has needs of her own or that having some needs is legitimate. As a result, she begins to form her identity around responsibility for caring for people, without being entitled to reciprocity or even recognition and acknowledgement. She may well develop pride in her considerable competence and ability to cope, but also in the mistaken notion that she has no needs. As an adult, a parentified child will tend to continue in these relational patterns.

Complementarities in the Couple Relationship

In families in which incest has emerged, the mothers of the abused children have usually been parentified as children. In young adulthood, they tend to marry men for whom (for a variety of family of origin reasons) caretaking is important. The husbands tend to be relatively dependent and immature, often with strong narcissistic or sociopathic features or exaggerated notions of entitlement. Frequently, the husbands who later abuse one or more of the children have had significant decrements or interruptions in the parenting they received, usually because of maternal depression, enforced repeated childbearing, or death. The fathers of these husbands have not been nurturant or regarding.

The couple develops a fine complementarity—she takes care of him, and that's fine with him. There is a pervasive lack of reciprocity in the dyad, but it is not totally unfair. She does obtain some kind of relationship on terms that do not challenge her uneven development. This type of complementarity is quite stable and can withstand a number of events. What it usually cannot withstand is the birth of children. The pregnancy and birth of the first child is the usual watershed event that destabilizes the complementarity of the couple.

The Watershed That Begins the Estrangement

Usually, the wife will attempt to lean on the husband during the pregnancy, and when the baby is born, will want for the couple to share at least some of the child care. But the wife is not very good at recognizing her own needs or negotiating for them, so she may send mixed signals.

In a family in which incest emerges, the husband has usually not responded, on any level, to the requests of his wife. He may resent her requests, the changes in the basic dynamic of the couple, and especially her decreased energy for taking care of him. He may already be sensitized to the loss of maternal caretaking and as a result resents the situation and her. The husband, either overtly or covertly, refuses to be there and take his share of responsibility, leaving the wife to her own depleted devices and wholly responsible for care of their child. (This family developmental model fits very well with the patriarchal model Herman [1981] found and analyzed, in which child care was highly gender related, with women expected to assume total responsibility and task functions and men relieved of both task functions and responsibility for raising children.)

Use of Resources or Worsening Estrangement

In a family in which the husband can tap into some resources to stop his flight and respond *on some level* to his wife, the probability of incest decreases significantly. Such resources might include support and reality testing from friends, insight on the husband's part, religious or subcultural affiliation that support male responsibility in the family, or determination on the husband's part to have a real family rather than what he grew up with. He may come to work complaining of fatigue because his wife made him take one of the early morning feedings, only to find from co-workers that they participated in child care at least to this extent, and that may shift his behavior and thinking. Or, because they now have a child, the couple may begin attending religious services that support the active responsibility and involvement of the father in the family as other than a patriarchal, removed figure.

The crucial element is the ability (or lack thereof) for either partner to change his or her old relational style. In incestuous families, the husband has continued to not take responsibility while continuing to make entitled demands on the wife. She, instead of actively dealing with this situation and claiming some legitimate needs of her own, gradually becomes emotionally and relationally avoidant. There is a great deal of cultural support for men to make entitled demands with no obligation to reciprocity and for women to adopt the sainted/martyred role rather than confront their husbands and take responsibility for her own needs. In such cases, economic considerations often enter into people's thinking.

In families in which incest has developed, instead of confronting the situation, the wife takes on a more passive stance and becomes avoidant of her husband, as he gives so little in return for all he expects to receive. Eventually, she becomes avoidant of her children as well. Many mothers of incestuously abused children report that they can relate well to children before those children learn to speak. It seems that during infancy, the mother can receive from her children because of the fusional nature of the relationship. But with the onset of the child's ability to speak, the relationship changes, becoming more social and calling for a stronger sense of self and those negotiating skills the wife never had an opportunity to develop. And so she distances herself, because for her, relationships take and don't give back. As this is occurring, the husband is becoming even more clearly relationally pursuant, because for him, relationships provide some of what he needs. He will tend to continue pursuing his wife, because he has always gotten from her, and also because he feels entitled to do so. He will also be relationally pursuant with some of his children to meet his own needs.

The Next Generation and the Inception of Incest

The situation becomes increasingly dangerous as the eldest child (usually in these families a daughter) begins to be parentified, and a second generation of parentified, depleted women in the family emerges. The mother parentifies the daughter around task functions, usually because the husband is not helping very much with tasks and the mother is depleted to begin with. The father parentifies the child around his needs for caretaking and emotional sustenance. Her siblings dislike and resent her, because they interpret the parentification as favoritism, and the family system devalues her anyway. The onset of incestuous abuse occurs gradually in a context of the mother's depletion and avoidance, the father's emotional neediness and self-centeredness, and the daughter's parentification and isolation within the family.

The incestuously abused child is in an extremely difficult situation. She is being sexually abused by a parent, with all this implies about the impairments in development I discussed previously. Her sense of confusion about her own reality testing, her relatively undeveloped sense of self, and the distortions in her object relations combine with a substantial trauma response. These combined factors leave any child in a poor position to figure a way out of this complicated abusive situation.

Most children have a very difficult time with the notion of disclosing. The problem is often one of deciding who they could tell. A child in this situation has very probably been warned and threatened by the abuser not to tell, as this might mean his incarceration, a divorce, or the breakup of the family, which he and the child would regard as the child's fault. She has no one else inside the family to whom she can disclose. Her mother is relationally avoidant; and, in any case, most incest survivors feel markedly cool toward their mothers. This seems to be in part because the child's mother has been relationally avoidant and usually unavailable for attachment. Also, the husband has usually not protected his wife's reputation to the children, and the girl's mother has not firmly established her relational stance with her children.

During all those years of family life, when most husbands and wives support each other in setting limits, defining boundaries, and setting examples, the husband in an incestuous family cheats. He makes the mother look like a prude or look unreasonable when she attempts to set curfews or guidelines for appropriate dress. He can be relationally pursuant to the extent that he will use unfair advantage. The wife, usually because of poor self-esteem and unacknowledged anger, does not counter this pattern. The upshot of course is that the daughter feels anger and contempt for the mother and is not in a position emotionally to use the mother as a resource. The mother is not easily forgiven for her emotional unavailability for attachment and dependence. The child cannot approach her siblings, as they will probably either not believe her, regard this as a sign of favoritism, and (as has actually happened in some families) rejoice in her misfortune. The person the child is closest to in the family is her father, but he is the abuser. Often the child will attempt to have him stop the abuse, but I know of no cases where that has worked except for a very short period of time.

In extreme cases of incest, as Shengold (1989) pointed out with regard to general physical abuse, the child's thinking partakes of the Stockholm syndrome. An abused person who has developed the Stockholm syndrome unconsciously bonds to the abuser as a survival strategy. If the family dysfunction is so severe that the victim is in the abuser's absolute power, the child can turn psychologically and emotionally for rescue and relief only to the tormentor, which makes for an intense need to see the torturer as good and right and to identify with the torturer. This would seem to be a more extreme version of vertical splitting. It implies that any sense of a separate self is compromised.

The full expression of the Stockholm syndrome is most usually seen in survivors of malevolent abuse (which will be identified as an important variant of the family constellation currently at issue). But many incest survivors show a mild form of this in their extreme protectiveness and loyalty to the abusing father and their fury at the avoidant mother.

And so the incest survivor that clinicians treat later, as an adult, has been a parentified child, with all this implies about uneven development and a poorly developed sense of the self. She has been chronically sexually abused—that is, traumatized—*within* her own family. She has grown up in a grossly distorted developmental context, which has distorted her experience and learning around boundaries, relational reciprocity, earned entitlement, uses of power, issues around nurturance, validity and recognition of needs, and even recognition of sensations, experiences, and reality testing. Her object relations are contaminated, and she knows far more about intimate betrayal than any of us want to. (This of course will complicate trust in later treatment situations.) She has become a stranger to basic feelings of security, safety, trust, and even nonvigilant sleep. Instead, in a field of emotional isolation, she is exploited, abused, terrorized, and treated with duplicity. She is utterly dependent upon the people who are doing these things to her, is still a child, and has no safe haven where she can run to hide, to talk to someone about things, or to be taken care of. Even a boxer has a manager and a corner to go to. The incestuously abused child does not, and she attempts to deal with all this through the protecting yet burdening haze of marked dissociation.

Malevolent Intent

These are the most frequent relational patterns found in incest. Things can get worse in a variety of ways, and the worst-case scenario is a relational one. That is when a child is being incestuously abused by an offender with malevolent intent (Gelinas 1991).

In most cases, the harm experienced by the child is largely peripheral to the intent of the offender, which may be a search for attention, affection, or nurturance; often, in fact, the offender will rationalize elements of the abuse to minimize in his or her own mind the extent of the harm to the child. Thus, some offenders attempt to explain things away by citing "a special relationship." This is clearly nonsensical and self-serving, yet it is also an attempt to not-see the destructiveness of it all on the child. Many offenders are uncomfortable with the issue of harm and so attempt to trivialize or explain it away. However, there are cases where the *intent* of the offender is to hurt, harm, and destroy the child. The trauma experienced by the child is central to the abuse for the offender.

The development of malevolent intent.   There is a deep and corrupted impulse on the part of some offenders to be cruel and to cripple or destroy the children they abuse. It seems to be an extreme end development of what Harry Stack Sullivan (1953) called the malevolent transformation. These are some of the cases in which atrocious things are done to the child target. It is an accurate way to identify situations where, for example, a parent repeatedly strangles a child to unconsciousness while sexually abusing her, allows the child to revive, and then tells her it will happen again, sometime that night. The intent is to terrify beyond bearing and to reduce the child to incapacity.

Although full consideration of the development of malevolence and malevolent intent is somewhat tangential to the present considerations, a brief look at its development will help considerably in understanding the dynamics of malevolence in abuse and its effects. It therefore makes sense to at least consider what Sullivan (1953) had to say about the start of the malevolent stance in life and relationship:

> For a variety of reasons, many children have the experience that when they need tenderness, when they do that which once brought tender cooperation, they are not only denied tenderness, but they are treated in a fashion to provoke anxiety or even, in some cases, pain. A child may discover that manifesting the need for tenderness toward the potent figures around him leads frequently to his being disadvantaged, being made anxious, being made fun of, and so on, so that . . . he is hurt, or in some cases he may be literally hurt. Under those circumstances, the developmental course changes to the point that the perceived need for tenderness brings a foresight of anxiety or pain. The child learns, you see, that it is highly disadvantageous to show any need for tender cooperation from the authoritative figures around him, in which case he shows something else; and that something else is the basic malevolent attitude, the attitude that one really lives among enemies—that is about what it amounts to. And on that basis, there come about the remarkable developments which are seen later in life, when the juvenile makes it practically impossible for anyone to

feel tenderly toward him or to treat him kindly; he beats them to it, so to speak, by the display of his attitude. (p. 214)

Those incest offenders who have focused on sadism and on inflicting the greatest trauma on the victim seem to be characterized by an endpoint development of the Sullivanian malevolent transformation.

These offenders often marry spouses who were themselves incestuously abused, and these spouses can become deeply damaged, oblivious, and sometimes collusive. One patient told me (and her siblings confirmed) that she used to sit outside the locked door of her siblings' bedroom when her stepfather was sexually abusing one of them, in the belief that her invisible presence would put some curbs on the stepfather's behavior and protect the sibling. On several occasions, their mother would tiptoe into the children's wing down the corridor to this bedroom, and my patient, when she was between the ages of 6 and 10, would silently take her mother by the hand and lead her back to the main part of the house. The mother did not intervene in the sexual and physical abuse of her children, and is only now, 30 years later, beginning to "remember" these events. In families with a malevolent offender, there may be one or two adults who were abused as children, no benign protecting adult, sadistic abuse, rampant dissociation, and duplicity across the family system.

Some effects of malevolent intent. Consideration of the development of malevolence as a stance toward other people is somewhat outside the scope of present considerations; the focus of my discussion in this chapter is on the effects of this malevolence on the child. Summit (1989) is right to insist on the centrality of the experience of victimization to understand and treat the survivor's problems: "In the absence of a trauma-centered conceptual framework and specific therapeutic interaction, the radical prospect of recovery and normality for survivors remains unrecognized" (p. 413).

Abuse with malevolent intent magnifies the trauma and the symptom picture exponentially, attacking the sense of self, the capacity for joy and pleasure in life, and the health, sanity, and sometimes even the life of the child. It can begin as early as infancy and continue well into adulthood, especially if the victim has developed a multiple personality disorder and one or more of the alters is compelled to continue visiting the malevolent offender. If the patient does not know this (and only one or more alters knows) and does not inform the therapist, it can be confusing for the therapist and dangerous for the patient. One patient realized after 6 months in treatment that she must be visiting her malevolent father because of unusual physical markings she was noticing on her body and money she could not account for.

These cases are not nearly as unusual as had been thought, and they continue to be underrecognized. It challenges credulity when someone tells us that she grew up in a family where the father repeatedly buried her before sexually abusing her; and when her grandmother became suspicious and confronted the father, he pushed the woman down the basement stairs, leaving her to die, and subsequently blamed the child to his wife, the daughter of the dead woman. One can only speculate what this might do to the mother-child relationship. Looked at from the perspective of individual psychology, how likely would it be that a child could have faith that anyone would believe her, or could afford to believe her? Could she afford to believe herself? One would think not. These malevolent developmental contexts are what characteristically produce multiple personalities among survivors.

All of this is clearly the worst kind of news. The good news is that most of what results for the survivor from such occurrences is very amenable to treatment, *if* the incest material is an explicit focus of therapy. Summit's point (1989) is essential here: there is a radical prospect of recovery and normality for survivors if, and only if, the clinical sequelae of these relationally based abuses are conceptualized and treated using the framework of trauma. The issues of what happened, and what effects they had on the child in the past and on the survivor in the present, need to be explicit emphases in therapy. The relational sequelae are an intrinsic part of this trauma picture.

Interventions for the Relational Sequelae of Incest

Trauma by a malevolent offender is a worst-case scenario in incest. It is an extreme variation of the basic individual, dyadic, systemic, and role-related relational patterns seen in practically all incestuous abuse. Even these basic patterns are difficult to change. They are multilayered, multidetermined, and interlocked.

These relational patterns are also highly tenacious. Incest survivors' families of origin usually continue to devalue and parentify the survivor well into her adulthood. Interestingly, the families tend to devalue the survivor in *exactly* the same ways, as well as using new types of devaluation and parentification; the relational patterns tend to be very rigid and mutually reinforcing. The families usually treat survivors as if they were still children in that family, with infinite obligations but no entitlement. One patient was flabbergasted when, at Christmas, one of her eight brothers poured a special cordial for each member of the family in turn and skipped her; she was 44 years old. This woman lived with several members of her family of origin and was not allowed to own a car or drive a sibling's car unless it was to drive other family members somewhere. When she attended religious services of her own choosing, the doors of her home were repeatedly locked on her. None of this seemed odd to her; it was sitting there in a circle of adults and being left out of the round of cordials that broke through her own denial about her family.

Usually, the adult survivor finds that not only does her family of origin continue to treat her unfairly in specific ways, but those in her current relationships also treat her unfairly *in the same ways.* She probably has few friends, and the friends she has may take unwitting advantage of her parentification. They may lean on her and feel closer to her than she feels toward them, recapitulating many elements of her relationships with her siblings. Her marital relationship probably recapitulates the unfairness in her family of origin; she may even find that her daughter has been incestuously abused by her husband, with her own avoidant relational stance contributing to the possibility. A survivor's children are often demanding and deeply disrespectful. The substantial changes she has made in her individual or group therapy is not recognized by those people in her current relationships and do not translate into relational changes.

Generally, changes from the individual therapy do not have much impact on the relational sequelae of incest. They do not seem to translate into the relational sphere for many survivors. This leaves them with internal, but little relational, change, which they identify as signifying only partial recovery.

Family therapy may have some impact on this, if used as a supplement to the individual therapy. However, it is not usually that efficacious as the only or primary form of treatment for incestuous abuse when the identified patient is an adult survivor. There are some inherent problems in attempting to work through the effects of incest by doing full-family therapy with an adult survivor and an abusive family of origin.

First, the family system very rarely has any motivation to change, or even to look at the long-denied abuse; families with incest are characterized by rigid and persisting denial. For most survivors, family denial is an important issue, but it should be dealt with only after the survivor has received considerable therapy. Exposure early in treatment to the family's denial is ill-advised. This denial can reinforce whatever denial the survivor may have, and it can also interfere with those survivors who are just beginning to regain memories and bring cognitive, affective, and somatic material back into consciousness. Attempts to treat adult survivors from the outset using family therapy would run the risk of exposing them to the family's powerful denial system prematurely.

Second, asking family members to come in for sessions can be problematic, because compliance and motivation are usually poor. Because the clinician is not treating a child victim, he or she does not have the kind of protective service leverage that accompanies work with an identified patient who is a child (Gelinas 1988). Compliance usually becomes progressively worse as progress on the family issues begins. When working with an adult survivor, family members typically drop out of treatment just when progress on the family issues is beginning; this, of course, is not coincidental. Third, the question arises of who will be paying for the sessions? Given the issues of entitlement, obligation, and devaluation that characterize families with incest, this can be a formidable question. Fourth, it is not unusual for the families to be superficially compliant but for the old structures to absorb and attenuate the therapist's efforts and never really change. These families can resemble the families of schizophrenic patients in this way and can be resistant to real change. The family therapist needs to be very confrontational and systemic and be knowledgeable about incest to be well-placed to do this work. Even then, it can be an uphill endeavor. Neither motivation nor leverage is present, and the therapeutic ally is the devalued member of the family.

Family therapy is usually most productively used as an adjunct to the adult survivor's individual therapy. Subsystem work can be quite productive as well—again, usually as an adjunct to the motivated individual therapy of the adult survivor.

An alternative approach is confrontation of the offender and the family by the survivor after very careful preparation with the therapist. This usually has fewer inherent problems.

Confronting the Offender—A Rationale

The survivor's confronting the offender is often very helpful, and sometimes even necessary, to correct old and existing relational imbalances. A thoroughly prepared confrontation can be the single most effective intervention I am aware of to change the continuing relational imbalances intrinsic to incest. It can operate simultaneously on a number of levels.

Confrontation is a direct power move. Although incest is an abuse of power, a great deal of the therapy addresses issues of fairness, intimacy, responsibility, and reciprocity. Confrontation with the offender both considers and corrects some of the power issues. Specifically, it challenges the misuses of power intrinsic to both the abuse and the relational structure of the family. It also reveals the secrecy and denial upon which the family has depended for so long. (Schatzow and Herman [1989] have written about adult survivors disclosing to their families, with the emphasis on breaking this secrecy.) Confronting the offender also challenges the fundamental relational structure of the family, because the survivor is refusing to occupy the usual devalued role in which she has infinite obligations but no entitlements. She is assigning responsibility for the abuse onto the hitherto overentitled abuser and claiming some entitlement of her own. This is where the responsibility should have been but wasn't until the confrontation.

Confronting the offender can also address and change some of the traumatic responses that were amplified by the relational basis of the abuse that I described previously. Residual doubts about reality testing, the nature of the attachment, the relation between self and other, and the locus of blame tend to resolve during the preparation and the confrontation. These issues are reflected in the typical content of the questions and comments the survivors wish to make, in the process in which they consider confronting the offender, and in their subsequent surprise at how much has changed within themselves and between themselves and others by this confrontation.

Part of the efficacy of this intervention, of course, resides in what it implies to the offender, the family, and the survivor. For an incest survivor to be able to confront the offender as part of her therapy directly implies that she has broken the secret—that she is *talking* about it with someone who is paying attention and believing her statements. This can be profoundly shocking to the offender and the rest of the family. It challenges the multilayered denial that has been central to the old functioning of the family, by ignoring the denial and *acting* on the survivor's own experience and knowledge.

Also, the fact that the survivor is taking the initiative rather than avoiding (i.e., asking for an appointment with the offender to talk about this material, and preparing to do so) implies that for the first time in her experience, *she* has mastery over this material. Before, she was mastered by the abuse, and it was used to control her; now she has control and is prepared (in both senses of the term) to use it. This is a classic situation of turning the tables, and it has a deep and lasting effect on the whole relational system and the survivor.

The confrontation can occur in one meeting or in several meetings between the survivor, offender, and other individual family members. The tone of the meeting(s) need not be brusque and offensive, but it should be firm and persistent.

It is important to realize that the benefits the survivor accrues from confronting the offender have almost nothing to do with how well or how poorly the offender and the family deal with the survivor or the confrontation, and almost everything to do with how well the therapist and survivor have prepared and how well the survivor is able to be there, confronting and hanging in there. That seems to be what transforms the survivor.

A particularly striking example of this point was a 20-year-old woman who I treated. She had significant brain damage from age 10, when a tree her father was cutting fell on her. She became entangled in the branches, and as the tree bounced as it fell, she was repeatedly slammed against the ground. She required 10 months of hospitalization and several surgical procedures for her extensive head, neck, rib, and leg injuries. It was during the subsequent convalescence, while she was bedridden in casts and a helmet, that the girl's father began pushing his penis through the bars of her bed and forcing her to fellate him. The idea of confronting this father initially appalled this woman, and she was faced with the ongoing problem of her poor memory and her difficulty in reading when she was anxious.

We prepared for 6 months and devised a written list with supplementary drawings to prompt her memory of topics she wanted to cover.

She made arrangements to see her father when other family members were either at work or outside working. When she broached the subject of her confrontation, her father got up and walked out of the room without saying a word. She had thought something like this might happen and had been prepared for it, so she simply followed him into the kitchen with her list and proceeded. He left the kitchen for another room, and she pursued him with her list and kept going. This went on for 45 minutes, at the end of which she had said everything she had wanted to say. Her father had not said a word to her, and she experienced her father, and herself, in an entirely new way. Within a month, on her own initiative, she had confronted her mother and one sibling, had moved into her own apartment, and was taking stock of her life.

Preparation, Residual Uncovering, and Resistance

The preparation for confrontation is very important and usually takes several months. It should begin with the therapist taking careful notes as the patient talks about old family interactions during the course of treatment. Often incest survivors have little awareness of how fundamentally unfair the family patterns and behaviors were, and they are usually a little confused about old events. Recounting childhood events and situations gradually clarifies these patterns, and the therapist should note them in the record and reflect this gently to the patient. These notes can provide a clear idea of the relevant issues for confrontation. As the patient gradually works through the traumatic material in the therapy and is clearly experiencing healing and recovery, the notion of confronting the offender can be introduced by the clinician, usually with a highly tentative question: "How would you feel if I said that I wondered if, at some point, it might make sense for you to confront your father/mother/uncle about the abuse?" The circumlocutions are designed to reduce the impact of the question, but often the response is shock and fear anyway. This response is striking and suggests how much work still needs to be done, which can be discussed, as well as how confronting the offender might help.

In this late phase in treatment, despite the considerable progress made in therapy, when the notion of confronting the offender is introduced, the depth of the survivor's fearfulness and the nature of her object relations with the abuser can surprise the therapist. It is not unusual for survivors to talk about the offender as if he were very large, a giant, or as though he might be a Godzilla-type creature (or a Medusa). This is a particularly good therapeutic opportunity to explore what appears to be a dormant and almost completely unmodified early relational introject. The extent of its lack of modification during the survivor's development can be quite striking. It has seemed that talking about confronting the offender has been the only reliable way to gain access to that early monster or giant introject in its full vividness. If for no other reason, the phase of preparing to confront the offender is important, as it allows work to progress on this abuser introject (or series of introjects). Additionally, of course, preparing and confronting accomplish other significant changes.

When the patient can tolerate these ideas, the therapist can begin the more direct preparation by asking her what kinds of things she would like to say to and to ask the offender. In point of fact, this is often a good question to help survivors see the possibilities in this confrontation idea. Then the therapist can help the patient make a list of questions and statements and ask her to carry the list with her to amend it as she thinks of things. This intervention is corny, simple, and remarkably effective. It makes the possibility of a confrontation feel more real. I ask the patient to bring the list with her to therapy and we work actively with it: "What statement or question would you like to lead off with?" "Why? What are you hoping to accomplish with this one?" And so on.

There are several common statements and question, such as "Why did you do these things?" "Why me, was it something about me?" "You are the one responsible for the abuse, not me." "You ruined my life/my childhood/my capacity to have sex with my husband." There will also be highly idiosyncratic comments relating to the particular history of each patient. This phase can last quite some time, as statements and questions are reworked. Also, the questions often prompt new material, which is then worked through.

Once this process is well under way, it is important to begin to work with the patient about how *she* wants to respond to each response of the offender. I will ask what she thinks the offender is most likely to say after she makes a particular statement or asks a certain question. Most patients will hesitate a bit at this, commenting that there is no way to know what anyone will say in any given situation. The therapist can simply acknowledge this, but then state that the patient has known the abuser for many years and knows what he is like. At that point, the therapist can ask the patient to speculate as to what two or three responses the offender might make to a particular statement or question. Once she has thought about it and figured out what some likely responses might be, I then ask her to think specifically how she might like to respond to each of these comments by the abuser: "If he does say that, how do you want to respond? What specifically do you want to say?"

I note to the patient that she does not have to come up with responses on the spot during the confrontation or with me, for that matter. She can figure out beforehand how she wants to deal with the offender's emotional, verbal, and behavioral responses, *before* she goes in to do the confrontation. This is usually a funny moment in the therapy. For most incest survivors, it is a revelation that they can plot and scheme in some fashion to get control in crucial interpersonal situations. During this preparation phase, for each statement the survivor will make to the offender, we work on two probable offender responses and how the patient wants to handle each of them. This prepares the survivor to be able to follow through during interaction and to not be squelched by the offender's usually automatic attempts to regain control.

Obviously, despite the most careful preparation, an abuser will say things the survivor did not anticipate. This has not proved to be much of a problem. If the patient is truly well prepared, there are relatively few surprises, and those are taken in stride, because they are occurring in a context where the survivor has managed to maintain most of the control. On balance, at the end of the confrontation, we hope that the survivor will have controlled the greater part of the interaction.

This preparation also uncovers material that has not been sufficiently worked through, especially around protectiveness and loyalty to the offenders and the family structure (Gelinas 1986). These patients are, after all, parentified individuals; for them, obligation to protect the family runs deep. The loyalty to the family should be explicitly respected by the therapist; the offender should be held responsible for the abuse, but the therapist must not scapegoat him nor allow the survivor to scapegoat him (Gelinas 1983). The offender is held accountable only for what he is legitimately responsible for and not necessarily for all the problems of the family. (Interestingly, the prospect of confronting the offender often acts as a corrective for those patients who are themselves prone to scapegoating the offender. Their loyalty and their tendency to scapegoat, which are usually kept compartmentalized and separate, are brought together, and a more realistic picture of the offender emerges. This can shift the survivor's relational stance to some degree.) Whole new layers of the survivor's felt responsibility also emerge and are now accessible for work, and these should be worked through. This often lends the preparation phase a two-steps-forward, one-step-back character, which, to me, seems unavoidable.

It should be emphasized here that the clinician can sometimes become impatient during this phase, as new levels of what can feel like resistance emerge to the patient's holding the offender accountable and to her moving out of the parentified role and taking the initiative in her own life. Frequently, the temptation for the clinician is to terminate the preparation prematurely and rush the survivor to confront, or to suppress (however subtly) the patient's reluctances and hesitations that reveal the deeper levels of her relational lack of entitlement. The preparation phase does not simply prepare the patient on a verbal level to confront the offender, although that is essential of course. It also creates a situation in the therapy in which the relational aspects intrinsic to incest are in the spotlight and can be worked through before successful resolution (i.e., the confrontation) can be reached. If a patient attempts to confront the abuser before she is verbally prepared with responses to his comments *and* has not worked through the internalized relational elements as well as possible with the therapist, she is likely to be verbally and emotionally overwhelmed by the abuser, who will then have neatly seized control of her once again.

The abuser's attempts to seize control can be brutally obvious at times: "Nothing like that ever happened, and no one will ever believe you. You've always been a pathological liar." In one particular case, because she had anticipated something like this kind of attack, the survivor had a written statement from her adopted sister describing her own sexual abuse by this abuser, and she confronted her father about his use of the term "pathological liar" as an attempt to divert her attention. During the course of this confrontation, the father was never remotely agreeable, but he no longer challenged the existence of the old abuse. The survivor's confidence in her own reality testing locked into place; she knew that she had known that the abuse happened.

Other attempts to seize control can be subtle. One stepfather when confronted by the survivor stated, "Well of course you'd want to talk with me about that. I've been waiting to apologize to you for years now. What took you so long?" Faced with this statement without preparation, it is probable that most survivors would experience some difficulty in spontaneously extricating themselves and seizing control of the conversation. Because she was prepared for something like this, the survivor actually began to laugh and noted his statement in writing, stating that that was exactly the kind of thing she'd told her therapist a person like him would say. He was nonplussed by her amused dismissal. She then told him that she would tell him what *she* wished to tell him, and he would listen; she was not interested in his apologies. She was interested in her own agenda about the old history of abuse.

Confrontation

When the patient is ready to confront the offender, she should make an appointment with him, for a setting that confers safety, and without having to be absolutely specific about why she wants to meet. This kind of confrontation should not be attempted, for example, on the way to the hardware store or at a Fourth of July family picnic. It deserves and requires the appropriate setting, which should be chosen by the survivor. Restaurants that provide some privacy work well, because they help to control the behavior of the offender, protect the survivor, yet provide some privacy. Other sites might include small public parks where there are people and shops, or a supportive relative's patio if the relative is at home. What should be avoided are all arrangements that leave control and safety issues in the hands of the abuser. Going for a drive in his car, meeting for a quiet picnic, going for a hike or boat ride—these kinds of situations should be absolutely avoided.

The patient can ask for an appointment to talk with the abuser about some important matters. If he presses her for details, this provides an opportunity for the survivor to practice hanging on to the control by simply stating that she will tell him at the meeting. If the abuser refuses to come to a meeting under those conditions, a variety of approaches can be appropriate. One is to say, "Fine, then I'll discuss all of this with my lawyer, your mother, my mother, etc." Another approach is to say that the survivor has been in therapy and wants to discuss some issues that have arisen; is there any reason he will not meet with her to talk?

It is useful to remind the survivor to bring the list to the confrontation. She will be anxious, and if her memory is impaired by her anxiety, she can have her list ready to refer to. I also ask that she bring her own tissues. She should not feel ashamed or defeated if she should cry during some parts of the confrontation; if this material doesn't deserve tears, I don't know what does. She just should not have to ask the abuser for a tissue or be disconcerted that she does not have one.

Usually the therapist should avoid participating in the confrontation. (I chose to attend confrontations if the patient is a child.) The therapist's presence at the confrontation would take away from the adult survivor's empowerment by implying that she needed assistance and was not up to this enterprise.

An important part of the preparation and the preconfrontation meetings is to remind the patient that the therapeutic benefits to be gained from this have almost nothing to do with how well or poorly the offender deals with the confrontation and almost everything to do with how well she has prepared in therapy and how well *the survivor* deals in the confrontation; that is, does she confront and hang in there?

If there are multiple offenders, she should confront them separately and begin with the *most* difficult one; usually a survivor will have only so much energy to do this and should accomplish the most important task first. If the offender is deceased, it is useful to help the survivor choose who, in the extended family system, is most responsible for maintaining an illegitimately benign reputation for the offender, and prepare for a disclosure or confrontation with that person about the offender.

If the offender has abused with malevolent intent, we examine if he has changed (occasionally some of them have had transformational experiences). If that change is pervasive enough, we attempt to evaluate whether contact with the formerly malevolent abuser will harm the survivor. Some malevolent offenders can be confronted, and others should definitely not be confronted. Some malevolent abusers may appear transformed, but when they are with the survivor, some old, corrupt part of their nature is revivified, and their contact with the survivor becomes malevolent once again. This should not be interpreted to imply that there is something about the survivor that elicits this on the part of the abuser; that would illegitimately shift the responsibility onto the survivor. Rather, there is something in some of these malevolent offenders that is triggered by certain characteristics in a large group of individuals, some of whom have been put into particular highly destructive forms of relationship with him, often by facticity. The survivor happens to be a member of this rather large group and one of the people in relationship in a particularly helpless situation. Then the therapist and patient need to find substitutes in the family system to approach and with whom to do this work. The presence of old malevolence requires caution and good judgment, though it does not necessarily preclude confrontation or the need for it.

When the survivor faces down her old abuser, the old power dynamic is stood on its head, and the patient—and the family—are different after that. She is claiming her entitlement—shifting responsibility to where it belongs, breaking the silence, taking control, breaking the old family structure, and staring down her old abuser.

Resolution

This intervention is a very powerful one, and a short period of mourning usually emerges as the survivor experiences the abrupt loss of her old childhood relational patterns in the family. The old relational patterns had in fact remained, practically frozen in time. This kind of confrontation radically changes them, so there is a sudden shift to the new adult status and the loss of the old child status. The therapist is in a position to help the survivor mourn this loss; get used to the relational, role, and self changes; and consolidate them. Having worked through the traumatic sequelae of the abuse and changed the old exploitative relational structures, the survivor is now free to begin building genuinely new relational patterns, and a life of her own.

References

American Psychiatric Association: Diagnostic and Statistical Manual of Mental Disorders, 3rd Edition, Revised. Washington, DC, American Psychiatric Association, 1987

Anonymous: Growing Through the Pain: The Incest Survivor's Companion. Park Ridge, IL, Parkside Publishing, 1989

Boszormenyi-Nagy I, Krasner B: Between Give and Take: A Clinical Guide to Contextual Therapy. New York, Brunner/Mazel, 1986

Boszormenyi-Nagy I, Spark G: Invisible Loyalties. New York, Brunner/Mazel, 1984

Ferenczi S: On the confusion of tongues between the adult and the child (1933), in Final Contributions to the Problems and Methods of Psychoanalysis. New York, Basic Books, 1955, pp 155–167

Gelinas D: The persisting negative effects of incest. Psychiatry 46:312–332, 1983

Gelinas D: Unexpected resources in treating incest families, in Family Resources: The Hidden Partner in Family Therapy. Edited by Karpel M. New York, Guilford, 1986

Gelinas D: Family therapy: characteristic family constellation and basic therapeutic stance, in Vulnerable Populations, Vol I: Evaluation and Treatment of Sexually Abused Children and Adult Survivors. Edited by Sgroi S. Lexington, MA, DC Heath, 1988

Gelinas D: Relational patterns in abusive families. Paper presented at the Psychological Trauma Conference, Harvard Medical School/Massachusetts Mental Health Center, Cambridge, MA, May 31–June 1, 1990

Gelinas D: Malevolent developmental contexts and transgenerational trauma. Paper presented at The Reality of Trauma in Everyday Life Conference at the annual convention of the International Society for Traumatic Stress Studies, Washington, DC, October 1991

Goodwin J: Discussion: malevolence, ritual abuse and sadism. Paper presented at The Reality of Trauma in Everyday Life Conference at the annual convention of the International Society for Traumatic Stress Studies, Washington, DC, October 1991

Herman J: Father-Daughter Incest. Cambridge, MA, Harvard University Press, 1981

Herman J: The treatment of trauma: incest as a paradigm. Paper presented at the Psychological Trauma Conference, Harvard Medical School/Massachusetts Mental Health Center, Cambridge, MA, May 31–June 1, 1990

Janet P: L'automatisme psychologique: essai de psychologie expérimentale sur les formes inférieures de l'activité humaine. Paris, Félix Alcan, 1889; Paris, Société Pierre Janet/Payot, 1973

Janet P: Problèmes psychologiques de l'émotion. Rev Neurol 17:1551–1687, 1909

Phillips A: Winnicott. Cambridge, MA, Harvard University Press, 1988

Schatzow E, Herman J: Breaking secrecy: adult survivors disclose to their families. Psychiatr Clin North Am 12:337–349, 1989

Shengold L: Child abuse and deprivation: soul murder. J Am Psychoanal Assoc 27:533–559, 1979

Shengold L: Soul Murder: The Effects of Childhood Abuse and Deprivation. New Haven, CT, Yale University Press, 1989

Sullivan HS: The Interpersonal Theory of Psychiatry. New York, WW Norton, 1953

Summit R: The child sexual abuse accommodation syndrome. Child Abuse Negl 7:177–193, 1983

Summit R: The centrality of victimization: regaining the focal point of recovery for survivors of child sexual abuse. Psychiatr Clin North Am 12:413–430, 1989

van der Kolk B, van der Hart O: Pierre Janet and the breakdown of adaptation in psychological trauma. Am J Psychiatry 146:1530–1540, 1989

Chapter 2

Group Treatment With Incest Survivors

Patricia L. Paddison, M.D.
Robin G. Einbinder, C.S.W., M.P.H.
Ellen Maker, B.S.
James J. Strain, M.D.

When we walk to the edge of all the light we have,
And take the step into the darkness of the unknown,
We must believe one of two things will happen—
There will be something solid for us to stand on,
    or We will be taught to fly.

Claire Morris

. . . only connect.

Howards End
E. M. Forster

*I*n this chapter, we hope to serve three purposes: 1) to outline and discuss group treatment issues with incest survivors; 2) to describe the group structure utilized at the Mount Sinai Medical Center; and 3) to present the results of a study looking at pre- and postgroup treatment measures conducted at The Mount Sinai Medical Center Rape Crisis Intervention Program in New York in 1990–1991. Although most of the theory and practice of group therapy for adult survivors of incest is applicable to both males and females, the following discussion pertains to adult female survivors. Sadly, the literature and studies of men who were sexually abused in childhood are sparse, and further exploration is needed as some treatment issues will be different. For example, because most male survivors are abused by adult men, sexual identity issues often arise as a consequence.

    The data on prevalence of sexual abuse that occurred in childhood among adult women ranges from 5%–62%. A national survey conducted with 2,000 adults revealed that 27% of the women had been sexually abused (Timnick 1985). In a random sample of 2,004 adult women in the community, Kilpatrick and colleagues (1985) learned that 14% of their sample had experienced sexual abuse. Another study in Great Britain of 2,019 men and women reported that 12% of the women had been sexually abused before age 16 (Baker and Duncan 1985). Russell (1986) surveyed a random sample of 933 women in San Francisco and discovered that 38% had been sexually abused before age 18. Wyatt (1985) found no differences in the rate of sexual abuse among ethnic groups in a study of 248 women in Los Angeles or among women of different economic status (Wyatt and Peters 1986).

Group therapy as an adjunct to individual therapy is recommended by many experts as an important step to working through the shame, stigma, isolation, and guilt associated with sexual abuse (Courtois 1988; Herman and Schatzow 1984). Time-limited group treatment offers many advantages. Herman and Schatzow (1984, p. 609) present three reasons for the efficacy of time-limited treatment:

1. The pressure of the time limit works initially to facilitate bonding and diminish the members' resistance to sharing emotionally important material;
2. It offers a structure within which the regressive aspects of treatment can be contained (e.g., the pain experienced when focusing on the incest has an endpoint); and
3. It permits a concentrated focus on the common theme of incest, with minimal attention to present differences and interpersonal conflicts within the group.

Additionally, Sprei and Unger (1986) list advantages of setting time limits for treatment (cf. Courtois 1988, p. 250):

1. Helps members who are only willing to make a time-limited commitment to treatment;
2. Promotes goal-oriented work;
3. Limits the level of anxiety experienced by a survivor considering joining a group;
4. Deliberately decreases the levels of dependency survivors can develop;

5. Provides a hopeful, optimistic outlook for survivors;
6. Provides a clear structure during the intense and disorganizing aspects of the treatment;
7. Encourages the emergence of feelings and issues that can be further explored in individual or long-term group treatment; and
8. Fits the needs and organizational structure of most sexual assault centers or other crisis service agencies.

Few studies have looked at the efficacy of group treatment in adult survivors of childhood sexual abuse (Alexander et al. 1989; Carver et al. 1989; Herman and Schatzow 1984; Roberts and Gwat-Yong 1989). Carver and colleagues' study of 95 women referred for group therapy for incest survivors showed significant improvement postgroup on the Hopkins Symptom Checklist—90 (HSCL; Derogatis 1983) but no significant change in self-esteem (measured by the Texas Social Behavior Inventory [TSBI]; Helmreich and Stapp 1974) or depression (Zung Self-Rating Depression Scale; Zung and Durham 1965; Carver et al. 1989). In a study by Alexander and colleagues (1989), efficacy of different types of group treatment was measured for subjects by the Beck Depression Inventory (BDI; Beck 1967), the Social Adjustment Scale (SAS; Weissman and Paykel 1974), the HSCL, and the Modified Fear Survey (MFS; Seidner and Kilpatrick 1988) against a control group. The researchers found improvement in both types of group treatment, especially the unstructured process group format. Many other studies reporting on subjective evaluations showed positive outcomes (Gordy 1983; Hazzard et al. 1986; Herman and Schatzow 1984; Knight 1990; Lubell and Soong 1982; Tsai and Wagner 1978).

There have been no studies looking at pre- and postgroup dissociative experiences or posttraumatic stress symptoms. Other studies have looked at depression and anxiety (Carver et al. 1989; Roberts and Gwat-Yong 1989) or also measured social adjustment, including marital adjustments (Alexander et al. 1989) or individual predictors (Follette et al. 1991).

Group Structure and Treatment Goals

Many variables need to be examined in determining group structure. Ideally, a group size of six to eight members per group allows time for each member to discuss her issues and to promote group process. Many times one or two members drop out, so careful screening to exclude clients who are not stable enough or motivated to commit to the group is important, because issues of abandonment can become exacerbated and disruption of the group process may occur. Precious time must be spent processing the loss of the member and allowing members a chance to explore feelings of abandonment. Also, despite a verbal contract and written guidelines asking members to attend one last meeting to say good-bye before leaving, many survivors are unable to do so. The remaining members are frequently angry as well as sad. An alternative strategy is to start with 8 to 10 members, anticipating 1 to 2 dropouts. We found $1\frac{1}{2}$ hours an ideal amount of time per week. Six months' duration allows group goals to be accomplished.

Two co-therapists are ideal and necessary to facilitate and process this difficult work. The co-therapists should discuss treatment (both structure and philosophies) prior to the start of the group, as well as allow time after each group in which to discuss the group process. There has been some discussion about whether the gender of the co-therapists is significant (Cole 1985; Courtois 1988; Courtois and Leehan 1982; Leehan and Wilson 1985). Most of our groups were led by women, with the exception of one group, which had male and female co-leaders. Some patients have a definite preference for female leaders because of their history of being victimized by men. However, having both male and female co-leaders may help to facilitate the transference process and play a valuable role in allowing the women to experience a man as caring and respectful of boundaries. However, Cole (1985) suggests that the primary task of incest treatment groups centers around the creation of trust, and the least threatening place to start may be trust building with women. Trust in men appears to come later. Clinically, it makes sense to give the patients a choice and to respect and support that decision.

Ideally, the group should consist of members who have completed approximately the same amount of treatment in regard to the incest (not necessarily duration but level of recovery). Dyads of similar background are preferred so that a member does not feel like the "only" one (i.e., not the only member who is an African American, Hispanic, substance abuser in recovery, homosexual, married woman, single woman, mother, etc.). Although this is not always possible, it is a vital part of the shared experience that promotes healing.

The goals of the group determine the criteria for inclusion of members, and the goals need to be related to the stages of healing. Herman (1992) conceptualizes recovery in three stages of healing. The first stage involves the establishment of safety. During this stage, biobehavioral strategies such as relaxation techniques, exercise, and meditation are helpful. Cognitive/verbal techniques such as lists, plans, and journals help to stabilize and promote self-reliance. Work on social strategies to promote support systems and reconstruction of a reliable attachment/relationship, such as self-help programs and individual therapy, are useful. The goal of this stage is to help stabilize and promote a "safe place" in which to proceed working on the aftermath of the incest in the second stage.

No attempts at in-depth treatment, either in individual or group therapy, should be attempted until the survivor is in a "safe place" emotionally and physically. Safety means no active substance abuse for many months, no active suicidal ideation, an ability to control impulses to self-mutilate, not being engaged in an abusive relationship, no recent psychiatric hospitalizations, and stability (not being in a state of crises) in the survivor's current life. During Stage One, Herman (1992) recommends brief (6–8 sessions) educational groups focused on relaxation and safety (not incest-focused) in addition to supportive individual therapy.

Stage Two involves reconstruction of the trauma. This work should not be attempted until safety is ensured. The locus of control (timing/pacing) remains with the patient. This process involves intense grief and mourning and carries a high risk of major depression. The incest work proceeds in small steps, and group treatment (time-limited and focused on the incest) is helpful during this stage. Here, the goal is integration of affect, memory, and cognition. The creation of some type of new meaning to life may occur.

Stage Three involves reconnection. This consists of the renegotiation of relationships within the family of origin, addressing the areas of boundaries, limit setting, and secrecy. The development of relationships, both peer and intimate, is important at this time. Social action and a "survivor mission" help transform and transcend the trauma by making it a gift to others (such as the telling of the story to others). To help address relational imbalances at this stage, regular group therapy directed at relationship issues (not incest-focused) may be indicated (Herman 1992).

The Study Group

The groups studied were time-limited and focused on incest. Members were in Herman's (1992) Stage Two of recovery, focusing on reconstruction of the trauma and attempting integration of affect, memory, and cognition. In describing the group structure, several case examples have been included. These are not specific cases but are composites developed to demonstrate the recovery process.

The first group meeting reviewed the philosophy/assumptions of the group and guidelines regarding confidentiality and absences. Written guidelines were distributed outlining the contract for attendance, missed sessions, and confidentiality. Contact outside of the group was not prohibited, but discussions were to be brought back into the group. Members were asked to tell each other about themselves in order to get to know each other and not to talk about the incest during this first session. The exercises and the basic structure for the next 6 months were outlined.

A volunteer was asked to begin the next session, to tell her story to the group and receive feedback from the group. This is done to decrease anxiety levels about speaking about the incest. Usually one member is comfortable telling her story, and it alleviates the rest of the group's anxiety about sharing their stories.

It was explained to the group that several weeks would be spent hearing members' accounts and receiving feedback from the group. The next period would be spent on members bringing in pictures of themselves at the age when the incest started. This exercise is a powerful tool to help members recognize their vulnerability and stop blaming themselves. Many women see themselves as "little adults," even when the average age at which the incest started was between 5 and 10 years old. The reality of how young and innocent they look in their pictures helped these women to stop blaming themselves. Also, looking at the pictures facilitated the remembering process.

Case Study 1

Ms. A had been sexually abused by the janitor in the building where she lived with her family from the time she was 6 until the age of 12. She had tried to tell her mother about the abuse when she was in second grade, but her mother had been unable or unwilling to hear what she was trying to say. Her father had been a prisoner of war, and the whole family spent considerable time avoiding "ruffling his feathers." Ms. A felt she had no right to "complain" further, as her family was dependent on her perpetrator's assistance (he performed many mechanical tasks for the family) and she felt certain that her father's suffering was greater than her own.

When Ms. A was asked to bring in a picture of herself at the age that the incest started, she stated that all of her childhood pictures were in her father's possession and she felt it would "upset" him to request the pictures. The group was able to point out that Ms. A had reverted back to her old distorted pattern of sacrificing herself for her father's well-being. Members also suggested that her view of her father might be distorted.

After prompting by other group members, Ms. A obtained the pictures from her father with no disastrous outcome. When she showed the group her pictures, she began to cry as she realized how young she had been to shoulder such responsibility for her family and how innocent a 6-year-old is, as opposed to her previous sense of responsibility for the sexual abuse.

The next exercise consists of the members writing a letter either to the perpetrator or the nonoffending parent, *not necessarily a letter to be sent.* This exercise is a tool to get in touch with feelings about the incest and as a way to empower their ability to be heard. Reading the letter aloud to the group and receiving feedback allows for further emotional expression that may have been previously repressed.

Case Study 2

Ms. B was an extremely insightful patient who had done a great deal of in-depth psychotherapy around issues of her incest prior to starting the group. During the first several weeks of the group, she was able to describe her incest and to experience many emotions surrounding it. However, when the group began working on the letter to the perpetrator or nonoffending parent, she was unable to write her letter, and she was the last member to bring one in.

With heartwrenching sobs, Ms. B read her letter to the group. She spoke of how the incest had not seemed entirely "real" until she put it on paper. She also admitted that she had not fully dealt with her ambivalent feelings toward her father (her perpetrator) and found it difficult to "confront" him in the letter. It was at this point that Ms. B was able to end a relationship with a married man who was emotionally unavailable to her.

We do not recommend disclosing to either the perpetrator or the family unless it is discussed thoroughly with their individual therapist and it is well planned. Many disclosures are disappointing to the survivors if their expectations are not met (Bass and Davis 1988; Schatzow and Herman 1989). Denise Gelinas, Ph.D., discusses disclosure and confrontation in depth in Chapter 1 of this book.

Case Study 3

> Ms. C shared with the group how she had previously confronted her father, who had sexually abused her as well as her siblings. She explained that she wanted to confront him when she felt in control so she would not be placing herself in danger, as he had been physically abusive as well. She volunteered to drive him home after he had had eye surgery and confronted him while driving 60 miles per hour on the freeway. She said that if he had tried anything, they would have both been killed. The group viewed this as quite courageous, missing the point that Ms. C could have been killed. This lack of concern for personal safety is often characteristic of survivors. This provided an opportunity to discuss ways of confrontation and disclosure and the importance of carefully planning all aspects of confrontation in advance.

The final exercise before termination consists of sexuality work based partly on the writing exercises from *The Courage to Heal Workbook* (Davis 1990). Specifically, members are asked to first write down what gives them pleasure. The second part looks at boundaries and asks members to list what is sexually safe, possibly safe, and unsafe. Many members requested work on sexuality, which is not surprising, as 78% of the women reported sexual problems at the time of the intake. Although these exercises were requested, there was resistance to completing them. In one group, not one member brought in the first completed writing assignment, indicating the degree of difficulty these women had in focusing on their own sensuality. Some examples members were able to list were listening to classical music, taking a bubble bath, and wearing silky clothes. Many of the women reported that it had been a long time since they had treated themselves to something pleasurable.

The second part of the sexuality exercise (listing what is safe, possibly safe, and unsafe) was even more difficult for group members.

The idea that they could define and set their own limits in having "safe" sex seemed revolutionary. This exercise became another tool to empower the survivors in setting boundaries and to give them permission to say "no" when specific types of touching are uncomfortable. (A more in-depth approach to sexual difficulties is outlined in Chapter 3 by Jennifer D. Bolen, M.D.)

This section provides a basic outline of how the groups were structured. These exercises helped keep the groups focused on the incest and also helped the process of connecting their memories with their feelings. The writing of a letter to the perpetrator or nonoffending parent seemed the most emotionally powerful exercise. Many members stated that it made the incest more real and helped them to get in touch with their feelings. Making the incest "real" involves not minimizing or denying that it happened and avoiding numbing their feelings about it. This process helped several members to begin restructuring relationships with family members in a new and positive way. Other members were able to sever ties with abusive family members. Some members actually sent their letters as a means of confronting their perpetrator or nonoffending parent.

The process of structuring and facilitating incest groups continues and changes with feedback from the group members and from other professionals. After the first set of groups, many members suggested more group structure focused on the incest. There are many ways to focus an incest group, but these exercises provided a format that we found successful.

Study Methods

We hypothesized that women with a history of childhood sexual abuse would show higher rates of dissociation, depression, anxiety, posttraumatic stress symptoms, and poorer marital adjustment. Furthermore, we anticipated improvement in these same symptoms after treatment in group therapy for 6 months.

Fifty-two women underwent a standardized intake interview for participation in a 6-month, weekly group of $1\frac{1}{2}$ hours during 1990–1991. The "Sexually Assaulted as a Child Inventory" (Jacobson et al. 1984) was administered as part of the initial intake. At the intake interview, the following psychological tests were administered: 1) the

Beck Depression Inventory (BDI; Beck 1967); 2) the Spielberger State-Trait Anxiety Inventory (STAI; Spielberger et al. 1970); 3) the Locke-Wallace Marital Adjustment Scale (MAS; Locke and Wallace 1958); 4) the Dissociative Experiences Scale (DES; Bernstein and Putnam 1986); and 5) the Impact of Events Scale (IOES; Horowitz et al. 1979). Completion of these forms was voluntary, and the women were instructed that acceptance into a group was not contingent upon participating in the study. The psychological tests were readministered at the last group session, along with a subjective evaluation questionnaire assessing the helpfulness of the groups.

The subjects were referred to the Mount Sinai Medical Center Rape Crisis Intervention Program in New York by other sexual assault programs and mental health agencies, through self-referral and community mailings, and by therapists. Inclusion/exclusion criteria were as follows:

1. In current individual therapy for at least 2 months;
2. No active suicidal or homicidal ideations;
3. Have memories of the abuse;
4. Stability in current life (not in a state of crisis or change);
5. No drug or alcohol abuse for the past year;
6. No psychiatric hospitalizations in the past year;
7. Motivated and willing to work in a group; and
8. Individual therapist confirms the above via a phone call.

The groups were free of charge and were facilitated by two therapists. The therapists were mental health professionals (psychiatrists, social workers, and counselors). Five of the six groups were facilitated by females, and one group was facilitated by a male and a female.

Study Results

A total of six incest support groups consisting of a total of 41 women were started in 1990–1991; 35 women completed the groups. Twenty-six women finished the group evaluation, and 25 completed the post-group psychological tests. A total of 56 women were interviewed for the groups, with 15 women either not meeting the inclusion/exclusion criteria or failing to show up for the first group meeting.

Demographics were compiled on the 41 women who started the groups. The mean age was 34 (± 10), and the mean number of years of education was 16 ± 2 (Table 2–1). Twenty-eight (70%) of the women's occupations were 5–9 on the Hollingshead Occupational Status Scale (A. B. Hollingshead, unpublished data, 1958). Fifty-nine percent ($n = 24$) were single, and 72% ($n = 28$) supported themselves. There was a fairly equitable distribution of religions, with slightly more Catholics than members of any other religion (38%, $n = 9$). Eighty percent ($n = 32$) of the women reported sexual problems (Table 2–2). Of the women with children, 78% (7/9) reported at least one incident of postpartum depression. Twenty-nine percent ($n = 12$) of the women had engaged in homosexual relationships.

Psychiatric hospitalizations were reported in 18% of the women

Table 2–1. Demographics of incest survivors starting group therapy; $N = 41$ (percentage)

Age (years)		34 ± 10
Education (years)		16 ± 2
Race[a]	White	20 (59)
	Black	9 (26)
	Hispanic	5 (15)
Marital status	Single	24 (59)
	Married	11 (27)
	Divorced	3 (7)
	Widowed	3 (7)
Religion[a]	Protestant	6 (25)
	Catholic	9 (38)
	Jewish	5 (21)
	Other	4 (17)

[a]Sample incomplete.

Table 2–2. Sexual problems in incest survivors; $N = 41$ (percentage)

Sexual problem	32 (78)
Desire	17 (45)
Arousal	11 (29)
Orgasm	14 (37)
Pain	11 (28)
Satisfaction	17 (45)

($n = 7$), and past suicide attempts were reported by 18% ($n = 7$). However, 63% ($n = 20$) reported past suicidal ideation, and 50% ($n = 26$) of the women interviewed responded positively to current suicidal ideation on the BDI. Past substance abuse (both alcohol and drugs) was reported in 36% of the women ($n = 15$). Family history of substance abuse was reported in 43% ($n = 16$), whereas family history of psychiatric disorders was present in 32% ($n = 12$). Thus, 75% of the sample had a family history of substance abuse and/or psychiatric disorders. Eating problems (specifically, being overweight) were cited in 58% ($n = 23$), with 10 women (25%) having binge eating problems and 2 (7%) admitting laxative use and/or vomiting in the past.

All of the women were sexually abused as children, with 11 (29%) having more than one perpetrator. Physical abuse in childhood was reported by 63% ($n = 24$) and in adulthood by 34% ($n = 13$). More than half ($n = 24, 63\%$) of our sample witnessed domestic violence in childhood, and one-third ($n = 12, 32\%$) experienced domestic violence as adults. Most of the women were abused by either their fathers or stepfathers ($n = 20, 60\%$; see Table 2–3), and almost all of the perpetrators were at least 20 years old ($n = 14, 83\%$). Ninety percent ($n = 34$) of the perpetrators were at least 5 years older than the victims.

Women were commonly between the ages of 5 and 10 when the incest began (Table 2–4). The duration of the incest was greater than 6 years in 56% of the sample ($n = 20$; see Table 2–5). The type of actual

Table 2–3. Perpetrator's relationship to survivor; $N = 38$ (percentage)

Father	14 (35)	Mother	1 (2.5)
Stepfather	6 (15)	Stepmother	1 (2.5)
Sibling	6 (15)	Friend	1 (2.5)
Relative	11 (27.5)		

Table 2–4. Age of victim when incest started; $N = 35$ (percentage)

≤ 5 years old	14 (40)	10+ years old	5 (14)
5–10 years old	16 (46)		

Table 2–5. Duration of incest; $N = 36$ (percentage)

6+ years	20 (56)	1–2 years	2 (6)
2–5 years	8 (22)	≤ 1 year	6 (16)

sexual abuse is reported in Table 2–6. Many women reported pressure to participate ($n = 20$). The pressure included physical threats ($n = 9$), nonphysical threats ($n = 10$), use of bribes ($n = 8$), and fearfulness ($n = 8$). As many as 43% ($n = 16$) stated that there were other incest victims in the family.

The psychological test scores at the initial interview demonstrated elevated levels of depression, anxiety, dissociation, intrusive/avoidant PTSD (posttraumatic stress disorder) symptoms, and poor marital relations (Table 2–7). Only 26 women completed the questionnaires at the end of the group. Surprisingly, posttest scores revealed that only the depression and anxiety scores showed improvement despite 88% of the

Table 2–6. Type of incest; $N = 41$ (percentage)

Intercourse	7 (17)	Oral sex	22 (54)
Molestation	27 (66)	Genital touching	26 (64)
Anal sex	4 (10)		

Note. These numbers are for those subjects who had only one perpetrator. Because more than one type of abuse may occur, these percentages add up to more than 100%. Also, 29% ($n = 12$) of the sample had more than one perpetrator; their data are not included here.

Table 2–7. Psychological test scores ($N = 26$)

	Pretherapy	Posttherapy	Significance
DES[a] (Norm = 4.4)	15	15	NS
STAI[b]			
Trait (Norm = 38.2)	54		
State (Norm = 39.4)	49	46	0.03 (−4.83, df = 23)
BDI[c] (Norm < 10)	19	14	0.008 (−4.42, df = 25)
MAS[d] (Norm = 100)	68	61	NS ($N = 7$)
IOES[e]			
Intrusive (Norm = 6.1)	19	18	NS
Avoidant (Norm = 6.6)	22	20	NS

[a]Dissociative Experiences Scale (Bernstein and Putnam 1986).
[b]Spielberger State/Trait Anxiety Inventory (Spielberger et al. 1970).
[c]Beck Depression Inventory (Beck 1967).
[d]Locke-Wallace Marital Adjustment Scale (Locke and Wallace 1958).
[e]Impact of Events Scale (Horowitz et al. 1979).

Table 2–8.   Follow-up questionnaire; N = 25 (percentage)

Respondents' opinions regarding overall group	
Helpful	22 (88)
Somewhat helpful	3 (12)
Not helpful	0 (0)
Damaging	0 (0)
Decreased isolation	15 (60)
Increased ability to trust	13 (52)
Less self-destructive behavior	11 (44)
Improved self-esteem	10 (40)
Less depression	10 (40)
Improved relationships with family	8 (32)
Improved ability to complete tasks	8 (32)
Improved relationships with significant others	8 (32)
Improved relationships with co-workers	6 (24)

group members ($n = 22$) stating that the group was helpful (Table 2–8) and the clinical observation that there were many positive changes. The follow-up questionnaire showed improvement in many areas, such as decreased isolation, increased ability to trust, improved self-esteem, decreased depression, and a decrease in self-destructive behavior.

The group members' scores on the IOES, which measures PTSD symptoms, did not significantly change over the 6 months, nor did those for the DES, which measures dissociation. The MAS scores did not show significant changes, but the number of women in relationships was low in this sample.

Discussion

This sample of women sexually abused in childhood showed elevated rates of dissociation, anxiety, depression, and intrusive/avoidant symptoms consistent with PTSD. It is important to note that the mean score on the DES was 15, with a range of 2 to 35. The literature reports that control subjects score 4.4, PTSD patients score 31, and patients with multiple personality disorder score greater than 50 (Bernstein and Putnam 1986). Dissociative experiences have been noted to decline with age and level off in the 30s (Ross and Ryan 1989; Ross et al. 1990).

Chu and Dill (1990) examined a psychiatric female inpatient group and found that 83% had DES scores above the median score of normal adults. Of great significance was the finding that 63% of this sample reported physical and/or sexual abuse. Sanders and Giolas (1991) examined a group of adolescents who had been psychiatrically hospitalized and found a significant correlation between physical abuse, sexual abuse, psychological abuse, and neglect, and elevated scores on the DES. We had hypothesized elevated scores on the DES in this population (group mean = 15) but are uncertain why the scores were not in the range for PTSD (31), whereas our IOES scores were consistent with PTSD symptoms. The DES may not be a reliable way to measure PTSD, or our stringent inclusion/exclusion criteria may have screened out the more unstable women. Also, the IOES may not be a reliable method to diagnose PTSD in this population, where the trauma occurred so long ago.

The fact that the group members' DES scores did not significantly change over the 6 months of sessions was surprising and is significant to clinicians in terms of efficacy of long-term treatment. If women tend to dissociate, they may be at risk for revictimization and may also have difficulty in working through problems in a relationship. For example, if a woman is in a situation that becomes dangerous, she may dissociate just at the time she should take protective action. An example of dissociation affecting a relationship would be the inability to work through an argument and reach resolution. Several of the women in our groups reported difficulty enjoying sex, because they would dissociate to avoid the discomfort of memories of incest. Other types of treatment, such as more focused abreactive therapy or cognitive-behavioral therapy, may be necessary to treat dissociation. In addition, it may be helpful to view dissociation as a defense mechanism that develops in childhood and that is difficult to modify after enduring childhood trauma (see Chapter 4 by Richard J. Loewenstein, M.D., for a more in-depth discussion of dissociative processes).

Lindberg and Distad (1985) reported on chronic and/or delayed posttraumatic stress disorder in a group of 17 adult survivors of incest. However, there have been no studies looking at PTSD in incest survivors pre- and postgroup. Our subjects' elevated scores on the IOES, which did not change after 6 months of group treatment, are disturbing. It may be that 6 months is not long enough to see a change in PTSD or dissociation, but most of the women had been in individual therapy for some time (56% for more than 1 year, and 60% in treatment more than once). It is possible that we need new treatment strategies to effect a significant change in these areas.

The decrease in depression and anxiety among group members is most probably due to the lessening of isolation through the group work and through forming new connections with family members. The catharsis for these women of telling their incest stories in a supporting, believing setting is not to be underestimated. Making new connections and learning to reach out for support were encouraged in the group. Many women went on to disclose to either their mothers or sisters and received validation and support there as well.

One of the problems of this study was the lack of control groups. The resources were limited, and offering treatment was a priority of the Rape Crisis Intervention Program. Many women had experienced childhood physical abuse (63%) and had witnessed domestic violence as well (63%). One-third of the sample went on to experience physical abuse and domestic violence in adulthood. Perhaps future studies should try to examine the women who manage to avoid further revictimization. In Wyatt and Newcomb's (1990) study on long-term outcomes of sexual abuse, the researchers found a close relationship between severity of abuse (type of abuse, number of abuse incidents, and amount of physical/psychological coercion) and degree of negative outcomes.

Better outcome measures and prospective, long-term follow-up are important to future studies. More stringent diagnostic evaluation for PTSD and dissociative disorders would help to clarify the role of self-rated tests such as the DES and the IOES. Finally, different instruments may be necessary to measure efficacy of group treatment.

Summary

Time-limited group therapy for incest survivors is an important component of treatment. The composition of the group, the group contract, and the participants' readiness and motivation to address the incest issues all play a crucial role in the treatment. Selecting patients at the appropriate stage in recovery is critical to minimize the risk of regression or decompensation. If patients are not in a safe place either physically or emotionally or free from substance abuse for a sufficient time, group treatment focused around incest may be harmful to them instead of helpful.

The amount of structure and the various exercises may vary depending on the therapists' viewpoint. The most healing aspect of the group treatment is the sharing and support that occur between members in a safe and dependable environment, resulting in decreased isolation and an ability to end the secrecy. It is important that the co-therapists discuss and outline treatment, structure, and philosophies before the onset of the group. Reviewing the process of the group after each session is essential for group continuity and also as an opportunity for the co-therapists to process any personally painful material. Any conflicts between the co-therapists will surely surface in these emotionally charged groups and need to be addressed promptly.

In conclusion, group therapy with incest survivors enables and empowers many group members to process their sexual abuse experiences in ways distinctly different from individual treatment. Many survivors become "unstuck" in their healing and are able to begin to address new issues, thereby transitioning from victims to survivors to thrivers. Many women were able to forge new and healthier relationships with their families and significant others; others were able to let go of the destructive, dysfunctional family/significant other bonds. The ability to heal themselves and each other enables the members to reach out and connect in new ways in their lives outside of treatment.

References

Alexander PC, Neimeyer RA, Follette VM, et al: A comparison of group treatments of women sexually abused as children. J Consult Clin Psychol 57:479–483, 1989

Baker AW, Duncan SP: Child sexual abuse: a study of prevalence in Great Britain. Child Abuse Negl 9:457–467, 1985

Bass E, Davis L: The Courage to Heal. New York, Harper & Row, 133–148, 1988

Beck AT: Depression: Causes and Treatments. Philadelphia, PA, University of Pennsylvania Press, 1967

Bernstein EM, Putnam FW: Development, reliability, and validity of a dissociation scale. J Nerv Ment Dis 174:727–735, 1986

Carver CM, Stalker C, Stewart E, et al: The impact of group therapy for adult survivors of childhood sexual abuse. Can J Psychiatry 34:753–758, 1989

Chu JA, Dill DL: Dissociative symptoms in relation to childhood physical and sexual abuse. Am J Psychiatry 147:887–892, 1990

Cole CL: A group design for adult female survivors of childhood incest. Women and Therapy 4:71–82, 1985

Courtois CA: Healing the Incest Wound: Adult Survivors in Therapy. New York, WW Norton, 1988

Courtois CA, Leehan J: Group treatment for grown-up abused children. The Personnel and Guidance Journal 60:564–566, 1982

Davis L: The Courage to Heal Workbook. New York, Harper & Row, 1990

Derogatis L: SCL-90-R Manual II. Towson, MD, Clinical Psychometric Research, 1983

Follette VM, Alexander PC, Follette WC: Individual predictors of outcome in group treatment for incest survivors. J Consult Clin Psychol 59:150–155, 1991

Gordy PL: Group work that supports adult victims of childhood incest. Social Casework 64:300–307, 1983

Hazzard A, King HE, Webb C: Group therapy with sexually abused adolescent girls. Am J Psychother 40:213–222, 1986

Helmreich R, Stapp J: Short forms of the Texas Social Behavior Inventory (TSBI), an objective measure of self esteem. Bulletin of the Psychonomic Society 4(5A):473–475, 1974

Herman J, Schatzow E: Time-limited group therapy for women with a history of incest. Int J Group Psychother 34:605–616, 1984

Herman JL: Trauma and Recovery. New York, Basic Books, 1992

Horowitz M, Wilner N, Alvarez W: Impact of event scale: a measure of subjective stress. Psychosom Med 41:209–218, 1979

Jacobson A, Richardson B, Simon J, et al: Physical and Sexual Assault Experiences Interview. Seattle, WA, University of Washington Medical Center, 1984

Kilpatrick DG, Bert CL, Vernon LJ, et al: Mental health correlates of criminal victimizations: a random community survey. J Consult Clin Psychol 53:866–873, 1985

Knight C: Use of support groups with adult female survivors of child sexual abuse. Social Work 35:202–206, 1990

Leehan J, Wilson L: Grown-up abused children. Springfield, IL, Charles C Thomas, 1985

Lindberg FH, Distad LJ: Post-traumatic stress disorders in women who experienced childhood incest. Child Abuse Negl 9:329–334, 1985

Locke HJ, Wallace KM: Short marital adjustment and prediction tests: their reliability and validity. Marriage Family Living 21:251–255, 1958

Lubell D, Soong W: Group therapy with sexually abused adolescents. Can J Psychiatry 27:311–315, 1982

Roberts L, Gwat-Yong L: A group therapy approach to the treatment of incest. Social Work With Groups 12:77–90, 1989

Ross CA, Ryan L: Dissociative experiences in adolescents and college students. Dissociation 2:239–242, 1989

Ross CA, Joshi S, Currie R: Dissociative experiences in the general population. Am J Psychiatry 147:1547–1552, 1990

Russell DEH: The Secret Trauma: Incest in the Lives of Girls and Women. New York, Basic Books, 1986

Sanders B, Giolas MH: Dissociation and childhood trauma in psychologically disturbed adolescents. Am J Psychiatry 148: 50–54, 1991

Schatzow E, Herman JL: Breaking secrecy. Adult survivors disclose to their families. Psychiatr Clin North Am 12: 337–349, 1989

Seidner AL, Kilpatrick DG: The Modified Fear Survey, in The Dictionary of Behavioral Assessment Techniques. Edited by Hersen M, Bellack AS. New York, Pergamon, 1988, pp 307–309

Spielberger CD, Gorsuch RL, Loshene RE: STAI Manual for the State-Trait Anxiety Inventory. Palo Alto, CA, Consulting Psychologist Press, 1970

Sprei J, Unger P: A training manual for the group treatment of adults molested as children. Rockville, MD, Montgomery County Sexual Assault Service, 1986

Timnick L: 22% in survey were child abuse victims. Los Angeles Times, August 25, 1985

Tsai M, Wagner N: Therapy groups for women sexually molested as children. Arch Sex Behav 7:417–429, 1978

Weissman MM, Paykel ES: The Depressed Woman. Chicago, IL, University of Chicago Press, 1974

Wyatt GE: The sexual abuse of Afro-American and white American women in childhood. Child Abuse Negl 9:507–519, 1985

Wyatt GE, Newcomb M: Internal and external mediators of women's sexual abuse in childhood. J Consult Clin Psychol 58:758–767, 1990

Wyatt GE, Peters SD: Methodological considerations in research on the prevalence of child sexual abuse. Child Abuse Negl 10:241–251, 1986

Zung WWK, Durham NC: A self-rating depression scale. Arch Gen Psychiatry 12:63–70, 1965

Chapter 3

Sexuality-Focused Treatment With Survivors and Their Partners

Jennifer D. Bolen, M.D.

*T*he purpose of this chapter is to discuss the experiences of working with adult survivors on their psychosexual functioning, both on an individual basis and in the context of an intimate relationship. Included in this discussion is a brief review of treatment for patients who have sexual difficulties, with a special focus on work with survivors of childhood sexual abuse. The challenge is to adapt a variety of well-delineated interventions developed for the treatment of the sexual dysfunctions to apply more effectively to this specific patient population.

Some of my focus in this chapter will be directed toward general sexual recovery at an individual level and/or in a partner context and will not focus solely on dysfunctions. General recovery areas included are healthier body image, changes in attitude toward sexual relating, assertiveness in communication pertaining to sexuality, and a better understanding of human sexual development. An example of one clinical treatment experience that combined group therapy treatment for female survivors and their partners will be described in more depth. The focus of this treatment was on recovery in the area of psychosexual functioning. This was accomplished by lessening the impact of the childhood sexual abuse on current psychosexual functioning. Issues related to the impact of the sexual abuse history on adult sexuality must be understood and carefully interwoven into the treatment.

The reviewed treatment and all clinical examples stem primarily from work done with female survivors. Some of the treatment experiences may generalize to male survivors, while others will not. It is important to keep in mind that this is a relatively new area of clinical work and is still in its early developmental stages. What is exciting about this area is that couples therapy, individual therapy, and group therapy techniques, both for general and for sexuality-oriented work, are highly evolved. Therapy developments in the trauma survivor field are also advancing at a rapid rate. This chapter addresses the integration of these bodies of knowledge to help survivors; this is a natural and, one hopes, successful step. Knowledge of all of the above areas should produce clinical approaches that provide improved treatment for survivors.

Historical Review

Contemporary sex therapy evolved following the hallmark work of Masters and Johnson on human sexuality and the publication of their books *Human Sexual Response* and *Human Sexual Inadequacy* (Masters and Johnson 1966, 1970). Sexual dysfunction training programs were offered across the country to teach students in the mental health professions specialized techniques for working with couples experiencing a range of difficulties in their sexual interaction. A major criticism in these early years of the Masters and Johnson approach was its potential for failure in couples with deeper problems. This was to some extent a conflict between psychodynamically oriented therapy and the more purely behaviorally oriented therapy described by Masters and Johnson. Psychodynamically trained therapists were skeptical that a structured behaviorally oriented therapy would produce lasting results for couples, especially if deeper problems were ignored.

Sex therapy was broadened by developing a more diverse and complex treatment approach with the publication of *The New Sex Therapy: Active Treatment of Sexual Dysfunctions* (Kaplan 1974). Kaplan continued to develop the treatment depth with her book *Disorders of Sexual Desire* and helped to integrate behavioral therapy and psychodynamically oriented therapy for the treatment of sexual dysfunction (Kaplan 1979). As she wrote, "A wide spectrum of underlying causes, varying in content and ranging from the mildest to the deepest and most tenacious, can be associated with sexual symptoms" (Kaplan 1979, p. 28). She goes on to delineate her definition of mild, mid-level, and deeper levels of anxiety that interfere with healthy sexual functioning. The deeper levels are associated with childhood injury and are often seen in desire phase difficulties. The types of injury were not outlined to any extent. In *Disorders of Sexual Desire,* sexual assault was given only the most fleeting mention as a possible injurious influence with a long-standing impact on sexual functioning. It would be a few more years before the field of survivor work erupted with publications and became a generally accepted area of clinical focus. The study of sexuality and sexual dysfunction as it relates to sexual abuse and assault has received growing amounts of attention (Becker et al. 1986; Jehu 1988; Maltz 1988; McGuire and Wagner 1978; Tsai et al. 1979).

Current Review

Literature on alternative treatment modalities in addition to the traditional format of sex therapy is currently in the early developmental phases with survivors of sexual abuse (Becker et al. 1984; Douglas et al. 1989; Jehu 1988; Maltz 1988; Maltz and Holman 1987; McCarthy 1990; McGuire and Wagner 1978). General texts on survivor therapy have had so much to cover pertaining to overall recovery techniques that often sexuality and sexual difficulties are given too brief a focus. In her excellent text on treatment designed for incest survivors, Courtois (1988) devoted only seven pages to sexuality.

Fortunately for many survivors and their therapists, the book *Incest and Sexuality* offered an excellent review of the impact of incest on sexuality as well as many ideas for healing (Maltz and Holman 1987). Maltz's latest book, *The Sexual Healing Journey,* offers couples a step-by-step approach to sexual recovery where one partner is a survivor (Maltz 1991). Additional survivor-focused publications include *The Courage to Heal* (Bass and Davis 1988), *The Courage to Heal Workbook* (Davis 1990), and *The Right to Innocence: Healing the Trauma of Child Sexual Abuse* (Engel 1989). Most of these general texts include a chapter on sexuality. However, publications specifically for clinicians have been sparse, whereas publications for survivors abound. At times the patients themselves are better read and better informed than their treating clinicians. Two excellent books aimed at partners of survivors have been released recently, and both have sections pertaining to sexuality: *Ghosts in the Bedroom: A Guide for Partners of Incest Survivors* (Graber 1991) and *Allies in Healing* (Davis 1991). A wonderful videotape, "To a Safer Place," includes some discussion related to sexual recovery (Shaffer and Turcotte 1989).

Another problem area in the field is the combining of prevalence data for adult sexual dysfunctions from different trauma groups (i.e., including survivors of adult assaults with survivors of ongoing, repetitive childhood sexual abuse; Becker et al. 1986). In the trauma field, the similarities and differences between differing groups of survivors has only recently begun to be studied. Negative and traumatic sexual experiences occur frequently in our culture for both men and women, and the lasting impact is at times quite subtle and less than apparent (McCarthy 1990). Psychologic resilience is often remarkable in overcoming past traumatic experiences, as noted in Herman's (1981) review of incest survivor responses. So many variables affect the short- and long-term impact of sexual assault that treatment orientation is by definition going to have to be individually tailored in most cases. There is much to learn regarding the long-range impact of childhood abuse on sexual functioning. Good prospective data on treatment outcomes for survivors are unavailable at this time. There are many interdependent variables that affect adult sexual functioning and sexual self-image. For example, cultural influences, developmental stage when the assault(s) occurred, severity of abuse, individual reaction and response, partner relationships, gender influences, family of origin, and many more variables too numerous to mention may all affect sexual functioning.

The feminist movement validated female sexuality with books such as *The New Our Bodies, Ourselves* (Boston Women's Health Book Collective 1984) and gave women a sense of ownership of their bodies. With numerous books on female sexuality such as *For Yourself: The Fulfillment of Female Sexuality* (Barbach 1975), women were given cultural permission to actualize their sexual selves. The movement for healthy sexuality occurred concurrently with the increased appreciation of the pervasiveness of sexual abuse in the female population. Prevalence studies on contact sexual abuse prior to age 17 revealed rates as high as 38% (Russell 1986) and 42% (Wyatt and Peters 1986) in the general female population. Of those women who reported abuse histories, 54% stated that the experience was "considerably or extremely traumatic" (Russell 1986). Survivors in recovery faced some painful contradictory realities between their emotional difficulties around sexual issues and the cultural changes regarding female sexuality.

Sexual Difficulties in Survivors

Several studies of abused versus nonabused women have noted a higher frequency of sexual difficulties in the abused group (Becker et al. 1986; Briere 1989; Jehu 1988). In Jehu's University of Manitoba series, 94% of survivors of childhood sexual abuse had at least one dysfunction, with the three most common being phobia/aversion (58.8%), dissatisfaction (58.8%), and impaired motivation (56.9%). Similarly, in another study comparing a nonassaulted group to an assaulted group, 58.6% of the assaulted group reported having at least one sexual problem, versus only 17.2% reporting this in the nonassaulted group (Becker et al. 1986). Furthermore, the types of problems reported were in different areas between the two groups, with the majority of survivor difficulties experienced in the early response-cycle domain, such as fear of sex, arousal, or desire dysfunction (Becker et al. 1986). The nonassaulted group that had problems in the early response-cycle domain experienced them in different ways, such as boredom with sex rather than fear of it. This was repeatedly correlated in other studies of psychosexual functioning in survivors, emphasizing the high prevalence of fear and aversion (Douglas et al. 1989; Jehu 1988; Maltz 1988; McGuire and Wagner 1978; Tsai et al. 1979). There was no difference between the two groups in the frequency of orgasm.

Many survivors report a lack of sensory input from the experience of orgasm as if psychic numbing, dissociation, or some neurological mechanism interferes. Some survivors report a noxious sensation during orgasm. Of interest, Becker and colleagues (1986) reported the occurrence of dyspareunia and vaginismus only in the assaulted group. This may be related to the smaller total number of dysfunctional nonassaulted women ($n = 17$; Becker et al. 1986) or to a significant relationship between prior assault and these dysfunctions. Women presenting with primary vaginismus and/or dyspareunia often are seen by non-mental health practitioners in primary care or gynecology settings and should be carefully evaluated for a history of assault in addition to their workup for physical pathology. A study of patients with pelvic pain showed a significant association between the presence of pain and a prior history of sexual abuse (Walker et al. 1988).

Sexual phobias are ubiquitous in survivors and often develop because of flashbacks or other aversive reactions that occur during sexual interactions. Flashbacks can be visual, olfactory, auditory, or tactile. These somatosensory experiences are common in survivors during sexual interaction and are usually triggered by any stimulus that evokes memories from past sexual abuse. The converse phenomena is also common: an absence of feeling referred to as psychic numbing, genital anesthesia, and other dissociative responses that place the survivor out of her body during touching interactions. At times, the avoidant and controlling behaviors that exist in survivors are often at an unconscious level. Even when the survivor is aware of the relationship between present and past, avoidance often predominates as a primary defense to intolerable panic or psychic distress. Loss of "here-and-now" contact occurs with severe flashbacks. Reliving the experiences can be such a powerful force that the survivor ceases to be present in the current reality with herself or her partner. She may avoid interactions that trigger a dissociative or reliving response as one strategy for preventing overwhelming abreactive experiences.

Sexual dissatisfaction arises if sex is perceived as dirty, evil, or disgusting (Jehu 1988), which are common attitudes in survivors. Many survivors view their bodies as contaminated, filthy, and disgusting; this especially holds true for their genitals and breasts. Sexual relating is an activator of these unpleasant and shameful feelings toward themselves. Often their dissatisfaction emerges in a committed relationship and has complex roots in the original incestuous family (Douglas et al. 1989). Because many survivors have a pervasive mistrust of men, over time they may interpret their partners' behaviors as similar to that of their perpetrators.

Sex Therapy With Survivors

Much of traditional sex therapy continues to be with couples and often works best for people who are partnered. The treatment is often symptom-based and less geared for sexual development and recovery of a wounded sexual self. Group therapy is not a frequent modality for treatment of sexual dysfunctions. There are some same-sex groups for specific dysfunctions, such as primary nonorgasmia and premature ejaculation. Individual therapy often works on sexual attitudes and beliefs, with some behavioral interventions for certain dysfunctions such as preorgasmia in females. With greater numbers of survivors being recognized in treatment settings and a growing body of information pertaining to more effective treatment, newer therapy techniques are being launched. Some of the creativity in trauma therapy stems from the reality that traditional psychotherapy techniques do not always work well with this clinical group.

Several treatment formats have been shown to be effective in addressing sexual difficulties in survivors. One study showed that group therapy was superior to individual therapy to treat the dysfunctions of sexually assaulted women (Becker et al. 1984). Other successful treatments have been couples-oriented (Douglas et al. 1989; Maltz 1988). Many women who seek help with sexuality issues do not have stable partner relationships, making it incumbent on the therapist to try individual therapeutic interventions or same-sex group therapy to address this area.

Adult survivors often spend years in individual therapy addressing issues pertaining to the sequelae of their child abuse histories. Many survivors at some point in their recovery process choose to participate in group therapy as part of their healing. Groups focus on the impact of the abuse on their lives in the "here and now" and also address issues of self-esteem, attitudes, cognitions, affect modulation, reactivity, and relationships. Often in general survivor groups, sexuality and body awareness are topics of focus, though the depth of this focus depends on overall readiness within a group of all group members. Survivors ready to work in more depth on sexuality need a specialized group where sexuality and sexual relating are the focus, with particular attention paid to the impact of their sexual abuse histories in this area of their lives. Because this area seems particularly affected by the taboo of silence, group members appear to give one another the green light to speak the unspeakable and break the taboo of silence. Shame and embarrassment remain powerful forces for silence in individual therapy but are often ameliorated in group through the sharing of their circumstances and the common human responses to their abuse. Prior to groups, many survivors view their responses as bizarre and somehow out of the range of normal humanness. Not all survivors are candidates for group, but those that are find the group experience rewarding.

Partners of Survivors

Partners of survivors are also affected with what are now seen as secondary effects. The partner's need for inclusion in the therapeutic work seems an important aspect of the treatment directed toward recovery of the survivor spouse and the survivor couple. Male partners often feel frustrated with their survivor partners' reactivity, avoidance, and aversive responses. Healthy partners are genuinely saddened by the abuse that their survivor partners sustained in childhood and are angry at the perpetrator. They often wish that their survivor partners would rapidly move beyond the abuse impact; therefore, they need the same interventions used with the survivor around the slow pace of recovery. Referring to the old fable of the tortoise and the hare emphasizes that it is direction and steadfastness rather than speed that allows for progress, growth, and recovery from sexual abuse. Additionally, though sexuality can be addressed rather readily in a same-sex group format for survivors, sexual functioning and dysfunction have traditionally been dealt with in a couples context (Masters and Johnson 1970). The treatment trial of the couples component discussed in the next section gives relationship work a focus, augments the survivor group work on sexuality and sexual relating, and integrates the two learning spheres.

Group Treatment Discussion

The following format for treatment of sexual difficulties in survivors is a time-limited group therapy model. Initially, the group was designed for the treatment of eight female survivors and their partners. Criteria for participation included a stable relationship as a couple, clinical stability with regards to self-safety, and no history of current substance abuse. Additionally, the completion of much general survivor recovery work plus a strong motivation to develop in the area of sexual growth were required. The eventual group size was half that originally planned and was thought to be more workable. The 4 survivors met weekly for the first 7 sessions of the scheduled 14, and then, after the holiday break, requested that they meet every other week. This better matched their treatment pacing needs, motivation, and time constraints.

The four male partners were seen once as a group at the beginning of the treatment sessions. They watched the 55-minute videotape "To a Safer Place" (Shaffer and Turcotte 1989), produced by a Canadian incest survivor. In the videotape, the narrator recounts her severe victimization history in childhood, interviews her three siblings and her mother, and candidly discusses her recovery process. Included is some discussion of her relationship with her significant other. The male partners had time after viewing this documentary to discuss their responses to seeing the tape and their reactions to sexual abuse in general and to their spouses' abuse in particular. They also discussed the personal impact of living with a recovering survivor. This first session was geared toward a didactic format and offered an opportunity for the male partners to bond as a group and to get to know one another as individuals before the couples' group sessions, which met once a month.

Two female therapists, both trained in traditional sex therapy, co-led the survivor group. A male therapist was added to the couples' group. He also had specific training in sex therapy. All three therapists were experienced, seasoned clinicians working with couples and individuals and had extensive clinical experience with patients affected by trauma.

The four survivors had all been in individual therapy for varying lengths of time. Two of the four had been in group therapy. One of the male partners had done some therapy for partners of survivors. The four couples all had stable, long-term relationships, ranging from a 30-year marriage to a 4-year marriage. Three of the four survivors were on antidepressants for treatment of clinical depression and anxiety. Beck Depression Inventory (BDI; Beck 1967) scores on all four survivors were in the nondepressed range.

A group flyer read by all the group members outlined the therapy focus and treatment modalities to be used in the group. Group members were all asked to read *Incest and Sexuality: A Guide to Understanding and Healing* (Maltz and Holman 1987). Additional survivor-focused publications included *The Courage to Heal* (Bass and Davis 1988); *The Courage to Heal Workbook* (Davis 1990); *Becoming Orgasmic: A Sexual and Personal Growth Program for Women* (Heiman and LoPiccolo 1988); *Ghosts in the Bedroom: A Guide for Partners of Incest Survivors* (Graber 1990); and *How to Make Love to the Same Person for the Rest of Your Life and Still Enjoy It* (O'Connor 1985).

Assessment Related to Treatment

An Index of Sexual Satisfaction (ISS) Questionnaire designed by Hudson and colleagues (1981) was administered at the onset of treatment and again near the end of treatment (see Table 3–1). Jehu's (1988) interview protocol for the assessment of sexual dysfunction was given to all couples. This was intended more as a vehicle for thought and discussion of sexuality development and sexual relating rather than as an instrument to fill out in its entirety. A Treatment Gains Questionnaire, developed by the treatment team, was completed by group members toward the end of the active phase of therapy (Table 3–2).

Treatment Phases

The initial five sessions of the survivor group treatment focused on individual sexuality. A physical therapist skilled in biofeedback and relaxation techniques attended survivor group 5 and taught the survivor group progressive muscular relaxation to use in conjunction with other anxiety management techniques to modulate fear. Anxiety has had mixed reviews in terms of its impact on sexual functioning. However, in general, it appears to be detrimental for most survivors, resulting in diminished interest, arousal, and satisfaction, as well as avoidance behaviors and dissociative responses.

Survivor groups 6–15 focused on problem solving on an individualized basis, including standard desensitization of phobic avoidance responses, changing reenactment behaviors, and pursuing treatment goals. Additional work on assertiveness for the survivors, especially in the interactional arena around touching and sexual relating with their partners, was a central assignment throughout the treatment. Interfering factors were addressed in an ongoing fashion and included a flare-up of

Table 3–1.   Index of Sexual Satisfaction (ISS) Questionnaire ratings

| | October 1990 | | April 1991 | |
	Survivors	Partners	Survivors	Partners
Couple A	56	18	33	21
Couple B	53	37	28	24
Couple C	29	14	17	16
Couple D	39	58	45	53

Note.   Clinical cutoff score for the ISS is 28–30, with less than 30 sorting out the "no sex problem" group and more than 30 the "sex problem" group.
Source.   Adapted from Hudson et al. 1981.

depression and panic in one survivor, a major loss for another survivor, and interactions with members of survivors' families of origin. Additional interfering factors are discussed in the next section.

Standard assignments for the couples included sensate focus exercises, both nongenital and genital. Various physical positions in part-

Table 3–2. Treatment Gains Questionnaire

	S1/P1	S2/P2	S3/P3	S4/P4
Comfort level has increased in your ability to communicate verbally about sexuality, sexual needs, and sexual concerns.	1/1	2/2	2/2	1/2
Able to speak up for yourself when relating to your partner sexually.	1/1	1/1	2/NA	1/1
Increased interest in your partner sexually.	1/NA	1/NA	1/NA	0/NA
Increased responsivity to your partner sexually.	0/1	1/1	1/NA	0/NA
Diminished aversion to being a sexual person.	1/NA	2/NA	2/NA	1/NA
Increased ability to separate sexual relating from abuse (to stop seeing sex as assault-related).	1/NA	1/NA	3/NA	1/NA
Improved body image.	1/NA	2/1	NA/NA	1/0
Less anxious and fearful when being sexual with your partner.	1/1	2/1	3/2	1/1
More comfortable with being a sexual person.	1/NA	1/1	3/NA	0/1
More comfortable with your partner being a sexual person.	1/1	0.5/1	3/NA	0/1

Paired responses (i.e., first response in each column is for first survivor and her partner; second response in each column is that of second survivor and her partner).
S = Survivor; P = Partner, Rating: 0 = No progress; 1 = Some progress; 2 = More progress; 3 = Much progress; NA = Not applicable or acceptable in the first place.

ner-related intimacy were explored, especially those that enhanced a survivor's sense of control and lessened feelings of helplessness. Body awareness work was predominantly a focus when survivors met without their partners. This included body image exercises, self-touching exercises, and education about human sexuality.

The initial couples group focused on communication styles and difficulties and on areas of previous growth and change. Subsequent sessions for couples continued to emphasize communication patterns within each couple and some of the shared understanding pertaining to living with a survivor spouse. Partners often understood the "tiptoe" effect of not bringing up the issues that would activate their survivor partners' distress.

Discussion

Over the 7 months of group, there were five major areas of focus in the treatment:

1. Separation of abuse from sexuality: cognitively, behaviorally and emotionally;
2. Integration of the male partner into the survivor's recovery;
3. Problem solving on an individual basis, such as desensitization formats, group support for change, discovery of reenactment patterns, and interruption of these patterns;
4. Need for control (emphasis on assertiveness); and
5. Interfering factors (depression, phobic avoidance, reliving experiences, stressful current life events, family of origin contact, and panic attacks).

These five areas would be active in any treatment pertaining to sexuality and sexual relating with survivors with or without integration of the partner. Further discussion of each of these areas follows.

Separation of abuse from sexuality. All four survivors experienced sexual problems related to the degree to which they were unable to separate their prior assault experiences from their current sexual interactions (i.e., thinking all sexual behavior was abusive or a violation of a person's body territory). One survivor was able to view her body and sexuality in a positive way. Of the survivors, she experienced the least dissatisfaction, both in her sexual relationship and toward her own body and individual sexuality. She experienced mild lack of sexual interest and lessened orgasmic response and frequency. She had additional factors impacting her libido and orgasm, namely a recent clinical depression and treatment for menopause and hypertension. Improvement in her general confidence level regarding open communication with her spouse resulted in much improved interest and responsiveness in the sexual domain.

Three of the four survivors experienced significant anxiety that was triggered by their partners. Triggering would evoke aversive responses such as physical withdrawal from the activity at hand, nausea, a sense of choking, disgust, and flashbacks. Different stimuli evoked these responses, including the partner's penis, sexual advances, ejaculate, breathing rate, smells, and kissing (especially French kissing). These three survivors had more difficulty separating their spouses from their abusers during sexual interactions. Techniques that helped survivors to separate the past from the present included turning lights on when having sex, having male partners verbalize during contact, changing position, letting survivors have control over the touching behavior and pace, and group support for reclaiming the survivors' minds and bodies from the past.

The first couples group was initially anticipated with fear and dread by the survivors, who spoke of coming into a room with unknown males as terrifying. Their experience in the first couples group was positive and the antithesis of their feared expectations, helping them to stay "here-and-now" focused. During an early couples session, all the participants practiced saying "I have a right to my own life" several times with increasing loudness. This exercise stemmed from the realization during the couples group of the degree to which survivors continued to feel controlled in current interactions and life decisions by their past conditioning. The constructiveness of the male partners and their humanness, sensitivity, and genuine respect was as healing an environment for the survivors as anything else about the treatment. The presence of nonabusive males in the group, supportive of their partners, went a long way in separating abuse from sexuality.

Integration of the male partner. The involvement of male partners in the therapy enabled the survivors to discuss their treatment with their partners. Couples actively supported each other in problem solving, communication enhancement, and risk-taking. A clear burst of hope and energy for continued recovery work followed each monthly couples session. The partners felt less in the dark and were better able to appreciate the vantage point of their spouses. At times, survivors were more likely to correct other male partners than their own spouses about misinterpretation of reactions and feelings common to survivors.

Many myths regarding male and female sexuality were explored and put to rest in this group. The presence of a male therapist in the couples group helped the survivors immensely in many general ways, but especially with a comment regarding male sexuality (i.e., that sex for males was not an emergency). All survivors had been conditioned to believe that men had sexual emergencies throughout the life span. The group was unanimous in their endorsement of the couples component.

Problem solving on an individual basis.   Body awareness work was particularly important to increase self-comfort and diminish self-phobias. One survivor was so phobic of her own genitals and breasts that her initial assignment was directed at breast self-exam, with an instructional card hung in her shower to help remind her of this important task. She had been chronically forced to massage her father as a child and had significant anxiety associated with her own hand movement when touching. Continued work in the area of self-touch was required and helped by a "reverse" hand-guiding technique. She felt less phobic with her partner's hand guiding her hand when touching her own body. She could experience significant arousal only in dreams and during sleepy times. Her assignments focused on decreasing avoidance to self-touch and using the Heiman and LoPiccolo (1988) guide to work on developing an orgasmic response. Having control of intimate physical touching was important to her ability to modulate anxiety.

Another survivor had problems with kissing, French kissing, and close face-to-face or ventral-to-ventral contact with her partner. Desensitization exercises to kissing and objects in her mouth were developed. Specifically, she practiced initially with a snorkel and mask in the bathtub, as she had severe anxiety with having an object in her mouth. She also had a sense of suffocation and nausea when her face was covered by water or by her partner's face. A nonsexual task using mask and snorkel worked to diminish her aversive response to these activities and transferred over to partner activities. She had no specific memory for her abuse, but oral assaults were strongly suspected. She was quite aversive to a male superior sexual position, which again left her feeling smothered and nauseated. Using the female superior or lateral position worked well for her. Practicing the male superior position outside of the bedroom helped desensitize her to this position (i.e., fully clothed, no sexual expectations, lights on, etc.). Daytime sexual relating also helped this patient. Lights on during touching exercises seemed to diminish the tendency to dissociate and experience the partner as a perpetrator. Looking at her partner's hair color and reminding herself that it was different from her perpetrator's were helpful cues to remind the survivor of her "here-and-now" reality.

One survivor read O'Connor's (1985) book, marking all parts of the text that applied to her. O'Connor writes about separating spouses from parents in the bedroom. This survivor was able to see that not feeling sexual toward her spouse helped her to differentiate him from her perpetrator father; this was an ingenious way of creating a new family that was differentiated from her family of origin. However, reexperiencing her partner as a sexual person meant that she had to develop alternative ways of seeing her current relationship as distinct from her childhood relationship. She worked on several assignments having to do with developing a sense of control and authority in relationship to her spouse. She also worked on seeing his genitals in a neutral rather than a negative way.

A helpful assignment for this survivor was to pretend to be a medical student studying the male genital anatomy, with her partner assigned to be an available model. Sexual relating was off-limits in this assignment. Also, this couple was given a prescription slip with the following assignment to help the survivor differentiate her partner from her father: 1) he was to request something sexual and she was to say "no" at least three times per week; 2) he was to react with distress and she was to hold her ground, working through her sense of guilt for not giving in to his nonverbal response to her refusal; and 3) finally, she was to remind herself repeatedly that his distress was not the same as her perpetrator's anger when she did not comply. During one group, this couple became aware of a pattern that seemed to reenact the childhood experience of feeling unheard. She tended to bring up important feelings just after bedtime when her spouse would be almost asleep; as a result, she would feel unheard. Also, this experience occurred at night at about the same hour as her childhood sexual abuse. She and her partner agreed to find alert, non-bedtime moments to talk and thus break this reenactment pattern.

Need for control. Over and over, the theme of the survivors' helplessness emerged in significant areas of interaction with partners. Continual work on assertiveness in general areas was practiced (especially pertaining to body territory and sexual relating) and problem-solved again and again. These survivors were skilled and competent women outside the marital domain but would often respond to spouses as if they had few or no rights. Their bewildered spouses all longed for their wives to behave in a more grown-up manner and often could not comprehend the degree to which their wives felt helpless in intimate relational patterns.

Interfering factors. Most therapies last long enough that intervening problems, stressors, and the like emerge to affect the recovery process. Depression and anxiety occurring in the context of treatment must be treated before sexuality work can continue. One member had a significant flare-up of low mood and panic. All survivors had issues regarding their families of origin that were current in their lives. Dealing with enabling mothers was a major focus for the group, and three out of four of the members worked actively on their current relationships with their mothers. The fourth survivor did more grieving for the loss of her mother during the group work when a favorite aunt was diagnosed with a terminal cancer. This aunt had also functioned in a mother role for this patient at a vulnerable time in her childhood.

One group member saw her perpetrator after some years of no contact. Her ability to stay self-oriented and protect herself emotionally in his presence was still compromised. Additional family work helped her to develop stronger self-protective responses and feel much more secure with her spouse sexually. Loss and separation affected two of the members. All such events provided more opportunity to develop skills that readily transposed to sexuality and the marital domain. For example, assertiveness with parents translated to assertiveness with spouses. Interruption of "exercises" by real-life events was a reminder that sexual relating is important, but never as critical as the maintenance of the self.

Summary

This treatment format was designed to provide survivors with an impact-oriented group experience. The group's focus was on sexuality and sexual relating but did not ignore the other domains of experience that affect the lives of survivors. These other areas included communication, assertiveness, family-of-origin work, and ongoing bereavement work. Overlap is obvious, because recovery in these other areas lessens interfering factors and enhances self-esteem, self-control, and self-mastery.

The integration of partners was a resounding success and lessened the feelings survivors had of alienation from men in general. It also gave a small amount of faith in the human race back to women who had had this faith desecrated in childhood. The couples component provided a unique opportunity for the survivors to work on the sexual domain of their lives as well as in their general recovery.

The interventions developed by Masters and Johnson and others were applicable to this group, with a more flexible and time-extended approach (Masters and Johnson 1970; McGuire and Wagner 1978). For instance, sensate focus exercises could be used intermittently throughout the course of treatment whenever a couple needed to drop back in their sexual relating because of survivor recovery needs or the reemergence of new memories, increased fear, and the like. Also, the concept of genital versus nongenital touching could be extended to practicing physical contact clothed or unclothed and to excluding any sexual contact when dictated by the emotional safety needs of the survivor. Traditional interventions are most effective when survivor reactions are understood in the context of their past assault histories.

Individual psychotherapy was ongoing for three out of the four survivors. This allowed them to work on desensitization formats, cognitive distortions, traumatic reactivity, and interfering factors in ways that clearly enhanced group work. The additional time for one-on-one interaction seemed to be helpful to process many feelings and reactions to the homework assignments and to address the interfering factors in more depth.

The Index of Sexual Satisfaction Questionnaire scores showed a clear improvement in three out of the four couples (see Table 3–1). The couple whose scores remained unchanged had significantly higher scores to begin with, indicating higher distress. This survivor had dominant interfering factors (i.e., depression and panic flare-ups) as well as burdensome family-of-origin issues slowing her pace of recovery. She had only recently begun to recall her history of victimization and did very well in this treatment, given the activation of an underlying posttraumatic stress disorder. She did respond with some positive changes in the Treatment Gains Questionnaire (Table 3–2).

The Treatment Gains Questionnaire showed progress for most survivors in the areas dealt with in the therapy. Survivors and partners all noted progress in their communication of sexual needs, sexual concerns, and general aspects of individual sexuality. Assertiveness with partners in intimate sexual relating also improved. Sexual interest and responsivity toward partners were areas with less progress. Survivors did show gains in being less aversive to accepting themselves and their partners as sexual persons. Furthermore, fear and anxiety levels for the survivors were lessened when they were being sexually interactive. Body image was better in the three survivors with impaired images.

The treatment of sexuality difficulties common to survivors and to their relationships is readily facilitated with a group format. The exclusion of partners in the survivor-only group component allows for greater comfort and freedom, enabling survivors to deal with individual aspects of their sexuality and to speak more openly about their relationship concerns. On the other hand, the inclusion of partners greatly assisted in the integration of partners into the recovery process of their wives and for themselves as couples. Sexuality issues were discussed quite openly in the couples group, in which they provided each other with much needed support. Partners consistently encouraged survivors to speak up for themselves and to see their perpetrators as separate from their partners. Communication between partners was significantly enhanced.

Obviously, the success of this treatment format is based on careful selection of stable couples and survivors who are well on the road in their recovery process. The addition of individual therapy or individual couple therapy for those needing more time may also be helpful. For the couple whose progress was slow, the timing of this treatment in the recovery process must be taken into account (i.e., it was early in the re-remembering phase, and the survivor was flooded with reliving feelings and reactivity). Time and a more focused couples therapy will most likely be helpful for this survivor. Integrating partners and spacing the frequency of sessions seemed sensible and helpful. The group also decided that the sessions would be extended from 14 to 20. Follow-up after the end of the active phase of treatment was to be monthly, alternating survivor sessions with couples sessions. Overall, this was a rewarding experience and a helpful treatment modality for survivors and their treating therapists.

Conclusion

Survivors are seen in all different therapy formats and many different clinical settings. Like most patients, they do not openly bring up their sexual concerns unless asked directly during history gathering. Because of their abuse history, they may be even more reluctant and at times overtly phobic to discussion of this part of their lives. Clinical sensitivity and good judgment about timing are an important part of helping survivors to begin to discuss their sexuality. Often the treatment needs for survivors are so encompassing that sexuality simply falls to a lower priority level as therapists and their patients attempt to cover more high-priority levels, such as self-safety, stability of mood and anxiety, and getting the survivor's life back on an even keel.

Addressing survivor sexuality is an important part of complete treatment for survivors and has clear benefits for improving their overall self-esteem, removing the stigma of difference that they feel pertaining to themselves as people, and enhancing their intimate relationships. For adolescent survivors where sexual abuse and assault affect the development of emerging sexuality, open discussion, responding to questions with available information, and (at times) a careful review of sexual development may prevent years of false knowledge and misunderstanding. One young assault survivor had worried for years that she was physically damaged by being raped at age 13. A general review of her current gynecologic functioning and permission to ask questions of her physician at her next pelvic exam led to marked relief for her. Psychological relief is also experienced by the older survivor who often has spent years feeling unusual in her sexual attitudes, responses, and reactions. Understanding the impact on herself individually and for survivors as a group lifts some of the burden of the abuse. Male assault survivors are often an unrecognized clinical group. With recognition, they are in need of the same careful review for the impact of their assault histories on their current sexual functioning and sexual self-image. With the increased appreciation of childhood sexual abuse experiences in males, clinicians might begin to look at rates of sexual dysfunction in this clinical group.

In conclusion, there are many rewarding aspects in the area of survivor sexuality for clinicians and their patients. This area can be approached with a variety of treatment modalities, including individual, couples, and group therapy. Traditional Masters and Johnson exercises are helpful, with a willingness on the part of the therapy team for imaginative alterations when clinically indicated, as well as skillful tailoring that integrates an understanding of the survivor's trauma history into the current treatment interventions.

References

Bass E, Davis L: The Courage to Heal. Harper & Row, New York, 1988

Barbach L: For Yourself: The Fulfillment of Female Sexuality. Garden City, NY, Doubleday, 1975

Beck AT: Depression: Causes and Treatments. Philadelphia, PA, University of Pennsylvania Press, 1967

Becker JV, Skinner LJ, Abel GG, et al: Time limited therapy with sexually dysfunctional sexually assaulted women. Journal of Social Work and Human Sexuality 3:97–115, 1984

Becker JV, Skinner LJ, Abel GG, et al: Level of post assault sexual functioning in rape and incest victims. Arch Sex Behav 15:37–49, 1986

Boston Women's Health Book Collective: The New Our Bodies, Ourselves. New York, Simon & Schuster, 1984

Briere J: Therapy for Adults Molested as Children, Beyond Survival. New York, Springer, 1989

Courtois C: Healing the Incest Wound: Adult Survivors in Therapy. New York, WW Norton, 1988

Davis L: The Courage to Heal Workbook. New York, Harper & Row, 1990

Davis L: Allies in Healing. New York, Harper Perennial, 1991

Douglas AR, Matson IC, Hunter S: Sex therapy for women incestuously abused as children. J Sex Marital Ther 4:143–159, 1989

Engel B: The Right to Innocence: Healing the Trauma of Child Sexual Abuse. Los Angeles, CA, JP Tarcher, 1989

Graber K: Ghosts in the Bedroom. A Guide for Partners of Incest Survivors. Deerfield Beach, FL, Health Communications, Inc., 1991

Heiman J, LoPiccolo J: Becoming Orgasmic: A Sexual and Personal Growth Program for Women. Englewood Cliffs, NJ, Prentice-Hall, 1988

Herman J: Father-Daughter Incest. Cambridge, MA, Harvard University Press, 1981

Hudson WW, Harrison DF, Crosscup PC: A short-form scale to measure sexual discord in dyadic relationships. The Journal of Sex Research 17:157–174, 1981

Jehu D: Beyond Sexual Abuse. Therapy With Women Who Were Childhood Victims. New York, Wiley, 1988

Kaplan H: The New Sex Therapy, Active Treatment of Sexual Dysfunctions. New York, Brunner/Mazel, 1974

Kaplan H: Disorders of Sexual Desire and Other New Concepts and Techniques in Sex Therapy. New York, Simon & Schuster, 1979

Maltz W: Identifying and treating the sexual repercussions of incest: a couples therapy approach. J Sex Marital Ther 14:142–170, 1988

Maltz W: The Sexual Healing Journey. New York, Harper Collins, 1991

Maltz W, Holman B: Incest and Sexuality: A Guide to Understanding and Healing. Lexington, MA, Lexington Books, 1987

Masters WH, Johnson VE: Human Sexual Response. Boston, MA, Little, Brown, 1966

Masters WH, Johnson VE: Human Sexual Inadequacy. Boston, MA, Little, Brown, 1970

McCarthy BW: Treating sexual dysfunction associated with prior sexual trauma. J Sex Marital Ther 16:142–146, 1990

McGuire LS, Wagner N: Sexual dysfunction in women who were molested as children: one response pattern and suggestions for treatment. J Sex Marital Ther 4:11–15, 1978

O'Connor D: How to Make Love to the Same Person for the Rest of Your Life and Still Enjoy It. Garden City, NY, Doubleday, 1985

Russell DEH: The Secret Trauma: Incest in the Lives of Girls and Women. New York, Basic Books, 1986

Shaffer B, Turcotte S: To a Safer Place. Studio D, National Film Board of Canada, 1989 [available from AIMS Media, 6901 Woodley Avenue, Van Nuys, CA 91406-4878]

Tsai M, Feldman-Summers S, Edgar M: Childhood molestation: variables related to differential impacts on psychosexual dysfunctioning in adult women. J Abnorm Psychol 88:407–417, 1979

Walker E, Katon W, Harrop-Griffiths J, et al: Relationship of chronic pelvic pain to psychiatric diagnoses and childhood sexual abuse. Am J Psychiatry 145:75–80, 1988

Wyatt GE, Peters SD: Issues in the definition of child sexual abuse in prevalence research. Child Abuse Negl 10:231–240, 1986

Chapter 4

Aspects of the Treatment of Dissociative Disorders in Survivors of Incest

Richard J. Loewenstein, M.D.

*I*n this chapter, I describe aspects of the treatment of dissociative disorders in adult survivors of incest. It is well beyond the scope of this review to provide a complete discussion of the diagnosis and treatment of dissociative disorders (for reviews see Braun 1986; Kluft 1988; Putnam 1989; Ross 1989; Spiegel 1991a). I will begin with a brief overview of the concept of dissociation and the clinical diagnosis of dissociative disorders. Discussion of treatment will focus on work with patients with multiple personality disorder (MPD), the most extreme form of childhood-onset complex chronic developmental dissociative disorder. A history of childhood sexual abuse has been reported in over 85% of adult males and 93% of adult females with MPD (Loewenstein and Putnam 1990). A history of incest has been reported in almost 70% of MPD patients (Putnam 1989). MPD patients usually report sexual abuse experiences that began before the age of 5 and tend to report the most extreme forms of repetitive, invasive, sadistic sexual abuse. Thus, this group illustrates many important issues in the treatment of adult incest survivors with dissociative symptoms. Similarities and differences between MPD incest survivors and non-MPD survivors also will be addressed.

What Is Dissociation?

Dissociation is usually understood in one of three ways: as a pathology; as a psychobiological process related to hypnotizability, altered states, and focused attention; and as an intrapsychic defense (Loewenstein and Ross 1992). Thus, DSM-III-R (American Psychiatric Association 1987) defines dissociation as a form of psychopathology in which there is a "disturbance or alteration in the normally integrative functions of identity memory or consciousness" (p. 269).

With respect to the second formulation of dissociation, Putnam (1991) states:

> Dissociation is a process that produces a discernible alteration in a person's thoughts, feelings or actions so that for a period of time certain information is not associated or integrated with other information as it normally or logically would be. This process, which is manifest along a continuum of severity, produces a range of clinical and behavioral phenomena involving alterations in memory and identity that play important roles in normal and pathological mental processes. (p. 145)

In terms of dissociation as an intrapsychic defense, Spiegel (1988) writes: "Dissociation has recently been understood as a defense not simply against memories of warded-off unconscious wishes, but rather as a defense against the traumatic experience itself" (p. 22). Kluft (1992) adds:

> Dissociation is pragmatically understood as a defense in which an overwhelmed individual cannot escape what assails him by taking meaningful action or successful flight, and escapes by altering instead his or her internal organization; i.e., he/she flees inwardly. It is a defense of those who suffer an intolerable sense of helplessness, and have had the experience of becoming an object, the victim of someone's willful mistreatment, the indifference of nature, or of one's own limitations; one realizes that one's own will and wishes have become irrelevant to the course of events. (p. 143)

Virtually all systematic reviews of dissociation note a robust relation between dissociative phenomena and traumatic circumstances such as wartime combat, natural disaster, concentration camp experiences, and interpersonal violence, including intrafamilial sexual and physical abuse (Gelinas 1983; Goodwin 1989; Kluft 1988; Loewenstein 1991a; Putnam 1985, 1989; Ross 1989; Spiegel 1990, 1991b). Spiegel (1990) delineates the overlap of dissociative symptoms and those of posttraumatic stress disorder (PTSD). Indeed, psychogenic amnesia is among the DSM-III-R diagnostic criteria for PTSD.

Following Ludwig (1983), Putnam (1989) enumerates a number of psychobiological functions of dissociation. These include

1. Automatization of behavior;
2. Resolution of irreconcilable conflicts;
3. Escape from the constraints of reality;
4. Isolation of catastrophic experiences;
5. Analgesia; and
6. Depersonalization.

It is not difficult to see the relevance to the understanding of the incest survivor of all of these formulations about dissociation.

Epidemiology of Dissociative Disorders

Systematic data are just beginning to be acquired about the prevalence of dissociative disorders in clinical and nonclinical populations. Recent studies of general population samples studied with standardized diagnostic instruments suggest that as many as 10% of the general population may have a dissociative disorder, including psychogenic amnesia, psychogenic fugue, multiple personality disorder, and dissociative disorder not otherwise specified (DDNOS; Ross 1991; Ross et al. 1990). According to Ross (1991), 1%–3% of the general population may have MPD. Similarly, using structured interviews and standardized rating scales for dissociative disorders in clinical and high-risk populations, Ross and colleagues have found dissociative disorders in 39% of patients in chemical dependency treatment, 13% of general adult psychiatric inpatients (thought by Ross to be a conservative estimate), 35% of a group of adolescents in psychiatric treatment, 35% of a group of prostitutes, and 50% of a group of exotic dancers (Ross 1991).

Dissociative symptoms are quite frequent in incest survivors (Briere 1989). In addition, the existing data support the clinical impression that more severe dissociative symptoms are associated with trauma that is more severe, repeated, and with an earlier onset. Thus, for example, Briere and Conte (1989) described a sample of 468 male and female clinical subjects with a reported history of childhood sexual abuse. They report that 59.6% ($n = 279$) of their subjects described an inability to remember the abuse at some time during their lives. Those with amnesia were more likely to have had more severe, early onset, repetitive, and physically injurious abuse with multiple perpetrators and direct prohibitions of harm for disclosure.

Diagnosis of Dissociation in Survivors of Incest

Dissociative symptoms can be grouped into several categories, including amnesia, autohypnotic, and "process" symptoms. The latter are most typically found in patients with MPD or DDNOS with features of MPD. Posttraumatic stress disorder, somatoform, and affective symptoms are also commonly found in patients with dissociative disorders (Loewenstein 1991b; Loewenstein and Putnam 1990; Loewenstein et al. 1988). For example, in a study of MPD and DDNOS patients at Sheppard Pratt Hospital, about 80% of the dissociative disorder patients met DSM-III-R criteria for PTSD (Armstrong and Loewenstein 1990; J. G. Armstrong and R. J. Loewenstein, unpublished data, June 1991). With few exceptions, the remaining patients had some PTSD symptoms short of the full criteria or had a lifetime history of PTSD that was in remission at the time of the interview. Virtually all of these patients gave histories of sexual and/or physical abuse in childhood.

Amnesia symptoms include blackouts or time loss, fugues, reports of disremembered behavior, unexplained possessions, inexplicable changes in relationships, chronic mistaken identity experiences, childhood amnesia and/or fragmentary recall of the entire life history, and brief ("micro") amnesias during conversations or other interactions with people. Autohypnotic symptoms include spontaneous trances, enthrallment, spontaneous age-regression, voluntary analgesia, negative hallucinations, depersonalization and out-of-body experiences, "trance logic" (a toleration of logical inconsistency characteristic of the hypnotic state), and spontaneous self-hypnotic behaviors such as eyerolls and eyelid fluttering.

Dissociative process symptoms include complex dissociative multimodal hallucinations and pseudohallucinations; passive-influence experiences; presence of distinct personalities or personality states; switching phenomena (i.e., transitions between these states); and linguistic changes, such as referring to the self in the first person plural or third person singular (Loewenstein 1991b; Putnam 1989). Dissociative incest survivors who do not meet the full criteria for MPD often have a mixture of autohypnotic symptoms, amnesia for at least some parts of childhood, somatoform symptoms, and PTSD symptoms. Anxiety and phobias will often be present as well. These are usually best conceptualized as a part of the PTSD syndrome. These patients commonly will meet diagnostic criteria for psychogenic amnesia or DDNOS with or without features of MPD.

All patients with a history of childhood trauma should be fully evaluated for chronic complex dissociative symptoms. Conversely, all patients with a history of dissociative symptoms should be assessed for a history of childhood abuse or trauma as well as for PTSD. The clinician should be aware that patients commonly conceal the presence of dissociative symptoms. Patients will hide these symptoms even from clinicians they know well unless a direct inquiry is made to uncover a history of dissociation. Thus, therapists of incest survivors should routinely perform a systematic assessment of dissociative symptoms. In general, the presence of such symptoms indicates a more severe childhood trauma history than had been previously expected (Loewenstein 1991b).

Case Study 1
(*Note:* All case studies represent composites of several patients.)

Ms. A came for consultation to assess the presence of a dissociative disorder after several fugue episodes. She had first sought psychotherapy after her marriage when she discovered that attempts at sexual relations caused her extreme panic. She had grown up in an intensely religious family and had no conscious awareness of having had sex before marriage. As psychotherapy proceeded, she uncovered a history of incest with an uncle when she was between the ages of 14 and 17. She diligently worked through these memories despite intense PTSD symptoms. However, she was still unable to have sexual contact with her husband without panic and flashbacks.

Next, Ms. A began to recall memories of being sexually abused by her grandfather from ages 9 to 14, when he had died suddenly and abuse with the uncle was said to have begun. She was hospitalized and continued to work with determination on these memories and her PTSD symptoms. Eventually these memories also were felt to be worked through, but the patient remained symptomatic. Her therapist reported that, at the time of consultation, the patient still had a complete amnesia for the first 9 years of her life. With direct inquiry during the consultation the patient revealed a lifelong history of time loss; fugues; disremembered out-of-character behavior; inexplicable changes in relationships; appearance of clothing, writings, and drawings for which she could not account; headaches; inner voices; passive-influence experiences; and autohypnotic experiences. The consultation revealed four alter personalities, one of whom described a sexual abuse history with Ms. A's father beginning before age 5. An even more complex childhood sexual abuse history involving several other family members was implied.

Treatment of Dissociative Symptoms in Survivors of Incest

General Considerations of Treatment

Basic issues in the treatment of the incest survivor with a dissociative disorder are the same as for incest survivors in general, although the dissociative patient may have even more complex and intense symptoms and posttraumatic transference reactions, as well as substantial hidden resources for recovery.

Difficulties around acceptance of the dissociative diagnosis, trust, boundaries, limits, dangerousness to self and/or others, establishment of a workable therapeutic relationship, and maintenance of the therapeutic frame are common in this patient population (Kluft 1991). Systematic approaches to these issues in the dissociative patient are described elsewhere (Braun 1986; Kluft 1984a, 1985, 1988, 1991; Putnam 1989).

It is thought that the therapist needs to be active, flexible, and "human" with dissociative patients (Kluft 1991; Spiegel 1991b). At the same time, the therapist must have a good understanding of appropriate boundaries and a clear sense of his or her role with the patient (i.e., as a psychotherapist, not as a public advocate, surrogate parent, detached detective in search of the "truth," etc.; Kluft 1991). The therapist must be able to set limits on behaviors that can undermine therapy, such as ongoing enmeshment with abusive individuals, severe eating disorders, substance abuse, intractable self-destructiveness or dangerousness toward others, and abuse of the survivor's own children, among others. Intensive work on childhood trauma should be limited until a safe space is created in the survivor's life by resolution of these sorts of difficulties (Turkus 1991).

A particular group of transference and countertransference responses regularly occur in the treatment of these patients. Usually, the transference is dominated by posttraumatic themes. The highly dissociative patient commonly experiences the world as a place where abuse is inevitable. The only freedom one has is to attempt to attenuate and/or manage the inescapable abuse. All people are perceived as potentially abusive or may be expected to violate boundaries with which they are entrusted, no matter what their official role description or reputation (Briere 1989; Loewenstein, in press; Spiegel 1986). Accordingly, the therapist is usually also perceived as potentially abusive and/or exploitative. Spiegel (1986) calls this the traumatic transference.

At other times, a flashback transference occurs in which the therapist is literally seen as a past abuser or other important past figure (Briere 1989; Loewenstein, in press; Spiegel 1986). In patients with MPD, some alters invariably are subject to flashback-transference perceptions. Alternatively, the therapist may be experienced in the transference as a co-abuser who is detached from and/or promoting of the abuse; as a failed past helper; and/or as the patient, with the patient taking the role of the abuser or of the therapist. In the latter case, the therapist often shares with the patient a profound sense of helplessness and/or impotence about the possibility of achieving any change or growth. The therapist must recognize this as a projective identification from the patient and interpret it as such. This sort of intervention may be successful in resolving stalemates in therapy resulting from such a transference/countertransference process (Peebles-Kleiger 1989).

A related process is that of the unconscious flashback:

> The individual has a sudden, discrete experience that leads to an action that recreates or repeats a traumatic event, but the subject does not have any awareness at the time or later of the connection between this action and the past trauma. (Putnam 1989, p. 237)

Unconscious flashbacks are very common in dissociative patients with a history of childhood sexual abuse. At some level, many of these patients may seem to be living in flashbacks much of the time. The therapist and the patient may unconsciously recreate old interactions between the dissociative patient and important past figures, abusive or not.

One of my patients called this "walking into the flashback together." This often painful process is related to the patient's psychogenic amnesia. The memories that make such difficulties comprehensible are dissociated. One tends to have the therapeutic predicament first; the solution to the problem only emerges as the amnesia abates, usually by uncovering additional traumatic material or by coming to a new understanding of previous material. In addition, some severe suicidal and self-destructive crises that occur with the derepression of abuse memories in incest survivors actually are partly related to the resurfacing of earlier suicidal or hopeless feelings that were dissociated at the time of the abuse. Clarification of this process level of the flashback experience may be a relief to the patient and may allow more successful resolution of difficulties in treatment.

Case Study 2

Ms. B was a highly complex dissociative patient with an extensive early history of incest with her father. She became increasingly angry, belittling, and taunting of me as therapy progressed. This process seemed to occur especially after some therapeutic gain or when she felt that therapy was helpful to her. At these times, she was very successful at getting me to respond angrily in return. She then was reproachful of me and herself. She stated that I often repeated the exact words spoken by her father in his interactions with her. This led her to profound hopelessness about therapy and our ability to work together. These difficult interactions frequently evoked similar feelings in me. Eventually I insisted that there had to be more to this pattern of interaction. Further, I stated that I could not be treated abusively by her any longer and that we had to resolve this process or therapy would be completely undermined.

Subsequently, Ms. B uncovered memories that clarified the interaction. When her relationship with her father had been loving and close, he had been more likely to sexually molest her. If she provoked him to anger, he was more likely to physically abuse her but less likely to sexually abuse her. Thus, in Ms. B's view, there were no other possible options in relation to a man. Clarification of this pattern was very helpful in reducing the frequency of these painful angry exchanges, in enhancing the working alliance, and in the patient's feeling greater freedom to respond in ways not determined solely by the abusive past.

Other countertransference reactions to the dissociative patient include exasperation, detachment, withdrawal, overidentification, and "secondary PTSD" (Kluft 1991; Lindy 1988; Loewenstein, in press; Putnam 1989). In addition, the therapist may experience depersonalization, amnesia, and other dissociative and trancelike phenomena in the intensely hypnotic dissociative transference field created by these patients (Loewenstein, in press).

Phases of Treatment

Sharing the Diagnosis

After the clinician makes a diagnosis of a dissociative disorder, it should be shared with the patient. It is useful to give the "official" DSM-III-R label, but to reframe the dissociation as an adaptive psychological process, not simply as a pathology. It is best to describe dissociation to the patient in simple, commonsensical terms. It is also helpful to describe concretely the relationship of dissociative symptoms such as amnesia and spontaneous self-hypnosis to the normal human response to trauma (Spiegel 1991b; van der Kolk 1986).

Many incest survivors with chronic complex dissociative disorders have an obsessional personality organization, not a borderline or histrionic personality structure (Armstrong 1991; Armstrong and Loewenstein 1990). Thus, they are particularly well-suited to an approach characterized by education about their disorder and support of intellectual defenses. Often these individuals have been bombarded by terrifying and perplexing symptoms that they usually interpret as a sign of "being crazy" or of having a psychosis. Although the diagnosis of a dissociative disorder may be frightening to the patient, there is frequently an admixture of relief as the patient begins to realize that there is a systematic explanation for what is wrong.

Similarly, if a diagnosis of PTSD is made by the therapist, it is also relieving to the patient to receive education about this disorder as well. Frequently, the patient expresses surprise that the symptoms of nightmares, flashbacks, intrusive imagery, amnesia, triggered panic reactions, and psychic numbing actually are part of a comprehensible clinical entity for which there is a clear method of treatment.

In discussing the meaning of a dissociative process with the patient, it is helpful to emphasize a number of issues:

1. Dissociation is an adaptive survival capacity meant to handle overwhelming experiences from which fight or flight was impossible.
2. Dissociation allows for compartmentalization of traumatic experiences so that the survivor could continue to develop psychologically as well as to preserve a capacity for relatedness to others despite the abuse.
3. The memories that are dissociated may be experienced as potentially very disruptive and overwhelming to the survivor. However, these memories have not been subjected to the "wearing away" that occurs with more ordinary memories, even painful ones. Thus, treatment must be allowed to go slowly to respect the inner "circuit breaker" system that the patient's mind has developed.
4. The dissociative patient is not so much "crazy" as adapted to a crazy childhood situation. The incest survivor with a dissociative disorder often describes a family characterized not only by abusiveness but also by a particularly malignant blend of severe sexual abuse, reversal of roles, loss of boundaries, and enmeshment in intense, confusing, complex abusive relationships, characterized by a double-binding mixture of torment and nurturance (Braun and Sachs 1985; Fine 1991).
5. Treatment does not involve destruction of the patient's inner survival system and skills. Rather, in the beginning of treatment, the survivor is encouraged to recognize, use, and modify dissociative defenses and coping capacities to help shape a more satisfactory contemporary adaptation. This is the beginning of gaining freedom from the legacy of the abuse that has heretofore determined much of the trajectory of the patient's life.

I conceptualize the treatment of the dissociative survivor as a collaboration in which the survivor is viewed as a resourceful person with significant health and strength. The dissociation is a reflection of this health and adaptability in the face of extreme, life-denying trauma. Actively working with the dissociation, rather than attempting to ablate or suppress it, empowers the survivor to move from a stance of feeling helpless, overwhelmed, trapped, and victimized (Spiegel 1991b). Utilization of the dissociativity of the survivor can help him or her reconstruct the past history to understand how he or she survived the trauma at the time of its occurrence. By so doing, the survivor can move from living in a perpetual flashback reality into a world characterized by greater freedom and continuity of thought, feeling, and action.

I usually share this view of the therapy with the patient. In addition, I attempt to give informed consent about the likely difficulties in attempting to treat a severe dissociative disorder. These include the certainty that the treatment will be intensely painful and that the patient will often be substantially more symptomatic for periods of time, even as therapeutic gains are made. The uncovering of hidden traumatic memories and their implications for the patient's life, as well as the relinquishing of dissociative anesthesia, make these treatments often exceptionally uncomfortable and distressing for therapist and patient alike (Kluft 1991). Nonetheless, the patient who successfully completes a treatment for a complex dissociative disorder is rewarded with a sense of mastery and freedom, coherence of sense of self, cessation of dissociative and PTSD symptoms, and real clarity about the meaning of his or her life history.

Reactions to the Diagnosis

Some survivors react more with relief than with distress at the dissociative diagnosis. Typically, these patients state that although they are upset at the label and its implications of severe trauma, the dissociative diagnosis is the first one that really makes sense to them and that comprehensively explains their symptoms and reactions. Although this acceptance is usually at an intellectualized level, these patients may readily begin to work in the dissociative framework to begin to explore more fully their current adaptation and past history.

More commonly, however, the diagnosis and the patient's reaction to it precipitate what might be called a "crisis of disclosure" homologous to that which occurs with disclosure of incest in an abusive family (Herman 1981). For example, in many MPD patients, there may be a stereotyped unfolding of alters with different perspectives about the revelation of the multiplicity and/or the revelation of the abuse history. Thus, some alters deny the MPD diagnosis; others readily admit the multiplicity. Some alters proclaim loyalty to the family of origin; others eschew the family or wish vengeance against its members. Some alters condemn the ones who have disclosed or punish them for revealing "the secrets"; those who have disclosed may feel overwhelmed, frightened, depleted, suicidal, and/or terrified.

Alternation of disclosure and retraction is common. Some alters fear that all will be destroyed by the revelation of the multiplicity. Other alters rationalize the abuse and/or personify the childhood abusers or co-abusers. These alters may insist that the incest was not abuse or that the patient caused the incest, deserved it, asked for it, should have prevented it, was helped by it, and so on. Other alters may describe complete bewilderment at what is occurring and/or disavow any knowledge or involvement in this "mess." Still others may respond by fugues, sexual indiscretions, or misuse of drugs and alcohol. At another level, the latter activities are often unconscious flashbacks that recreate aspects of the abuse that occurred in the patient's past and/or reflect attempts by the patient to control the emerging memories of trauma.

Severely dissociative incest survivors without MPD may show a similar set of conflicts and a sense of inner division and fragmentation over the disclosure of the dissociative process and/or the incest history, but without the florid multiplicity. In either case, overt PTSD may become manifest or may become exacerbated as deeper levels of disclosure occur. Patients commonly become more symptomatic with flashbacks, nightmares, acute amnesias, fugues, trances, somatoform symptoms, and panic. Suicidal and self-destructive crises are common at this point in treatment. Both therapist and patient may doubt the wisdom of proceeding further; frequently, there is a wish to "seal over" the patient by using suppressive interventions. Once the dissociative process begins to unfold, however, this is usually not a workable option.

However, there are supportive methods to help weather this storm and to help the patient achieve a more stable adaptation that permits treatment to go forward. First, the therapist must be aware that it is possible to work through such crises successfully, although usually only with consistent therapeutic work over a period of time.

It is important for the therapist to remain evenhanded and balanced as this highly conflictual material emerges (Putnam 1989; Kluft 1991). If the patient has MPD, the therapist must not play favorites in the battles between the alters, reframing that each one represents an attempt to help and handle some aspect of the abusive childhood experiences. Each alter must be heard, understood, and worked with systematically. Indeed, it is often the angry and/or persecutory alters that contain the most inherent positive life force. They are usually the staunchest helpers once enlisted in the service of the therapy.

For the non-MPD incest survivor with dissociative symptoms, a similar stance is important. The survivor may have very complex feelings and relationships with abusers and other family members. In general, it is helpful for the therapist to understand that dissociated material is likely to be "layered" and will not emerge all at once (Kluft 1984b; Putnam 1989). Often the survivor's understanding of the role of family members in the abuse will change as treatment progresses and more dissociative memory gaps are undone. Thus, the therapist should encourage all points of view about the past history to emerge. The survivor has the ultimate task of resolving the conflictual or contradictory feelings about abusers, other past figures, and past events. This occurs with the therapist's collaboration and consultation but is not ultimately determined by the therapist. On the other hand, the therapist should not hesitate to be a firm advocate of nonabusive values; he or she should challenge rationalizations of abusive behavior either in the patient's past or current life. At these times, it is often helpful to call the survivor's attention to the contradictory ways that he or she has described abusive people or to obvious dissociation of idea and affect in discussing important others (Fine 1991).

It is helpful to take a "systems" approach to the severely dissociative patient in whom so much information is compartmentalized and hidden. For example, in an MPD patient, the "personality" of the patient is really the sum of all the patient's alternate personalities. The patient is the whole human being, not simply the "host" personality or the one that carries the patient's legal name. No alter is more "real" than any other, and each plays a crucial role in the therapy. Attempts by "nice" personalities to suppress the emergence of angry, persecutory, self-destructive, and/or dysfunctional alters may represent the suppressive, controlling, authoritarian style of the incest family just as much as the alters who urge harm to the body as a punishment for revelation of the secrets. Often the latter are secret protectors who style themselves after abusers as protective coloration.

Case Study 3

Ms. C, a patient with known MPD, was hospitalized because of recurrent self-mutilation, insertion of knives into her vagina, panic attacks, and fugues. She described a history of sexual abuse beginning at age 3 involving repeated incestuous rape by her father, who was a fundamentalist Christian. Her outpatient therapist had refused to speak with the male alter that claimed responsibility for the self-destructive acts, stating she would "give him a dose of his own medicine." Two frightened, traumatized child alters kept emerging at work, disrupting the patient's employment. Another alter was "very religious" and maintained allegiance to the patient's father, calling him over the objections of the others.

The host personality spent considerable energy in attempting to suppress, ignore, and extirpate the other alters. When Ms. C was in the hospital, the host was encouraged to listen to the others. They were given a chance to speak if they agreed to stop self-destructive behavior. The host very reluctantly agreed. The male alter ultimately described himself as a sort of guerrilla protector who had been able to control the father's abusiveness by acting "crazy" during the abuse. The father was apparently dissuaded from attacking her as frequently when the patient actually appeared completely out of control. The alter was responsive to reframing his activities as similar to those of a combat veteran who continues to wear fatigues and carry weapons as if the war had not yet ended. He agreed to suspend self-destructive actions if he could be heard and comforted by the others. The religious alter agreed to suspend calls to the father.

The therapist suggested to the host alter that suppression and control are not the same. Real control would come from increasing awareness of the other alters, working directly with them and attempting to accept the memories, thoughts, and feelings that they contained. Suppression of them was a sort of mental apartheid that could only result in internal warfare and guerrilla activity. Ms. C was taught self-hypnotic techniques for symptom control (see next section). After Ms. C's discharge from the hospital and transfer to a new therapist, the alters were more able to communicate together and act adaptively. Self-destructive and dysfunctional behavior was significantly less, although substantial difficulties remained, primarily in Ms. C's relationships with her husband and children.

Supportive Interventions for Dissociative Symptoms

In the long-term outpatient psychotherapy of the dissociative incest survivor, it is important that the therapist help pace and structure the intensity of the treatment. The returning dissociated memories can act as a virtual phobic stimulus, with the patient feeling intensely flooded, terrified, helpless, out of control, and overwhelmed by an explosion of triggered flashbacks and spontaneous abreactions. At a process level, this phenomena parallels the patient's actual childhood experiences. In childhood, the patient usually felt helpless to prevent the abuse, was continually bombarded by abusive experiences, and felt unable to find respite. It is important to help the patient with the experience of being flooded, because, as Kluft (1991) points out, once the survivor's therapy feels unpredictable and/or unsafe, the whole endeavor may be markedly prolonged.

It may be helpful to the patient simply to understand the parallel process with the original experiences as a way of taking some distance from what is occurring. More concretely, it is useful for the therapist to educate the patient about the need to "separate time" (i.e., to use simple cognitive techniques to attempt to distance from a situation). For example, the patient may ask him- or herself: "Is this really another abusive situation, or is it simply one that has similar elements that trigger me into a flashback?" One patient paraphrased this as: "Is it real or is it Memorex?"

Dissociative patients can use their well-developed self-observing capacities to work on this sort of problem. Because so many of these patients' triggers are interpersonal, the therapy itself can be an important laboratory for examining the stimuli that bring on flashbacks. The dissociative survivor may need to prompt him- or herself continually outside of sessions to stay oriented to current reality. Some MPD patients literally post reminders of the current date and place in their homes so alters who are "lost" in perpetual flashbacks can orient to contemporary reality.

This process of examining reactions to triggers also encourages a beginning sense of freedom of thought and of choice in the survivor. The flashback response is automatic and intensely compelling; it does not permit the survivor to decide freely whether a situation or a person is abusive or not. This can only come with the ability to know the difference between the abusive past and contemporary reality, with all of its ambiguities and complexity. The idea of free choice may seem quite novel to the highly dissociative patient. He or she is usually skeptical that free choice exists in any way. This is one of the many cognitive distortions that permeate the survivor's thinking. Systematic work on this and other cognitive distortions is a crucial part of the therapy of the dissociative incest survivor (Fine 1988, 1990, 1991).

In a patient with very complex dissociative amnesia, it may be more helpful to achieve an intellectualized, cognitive overview of the patient's life before entering into intense abreactive work. This notion is summarized aptly by Yogi Berra, who once said: "You have to be careful if you don't know where you're going, because you might not get there."

Several interventions are useful to achieve an attenuation of affect for returning dissociated memories. If the patient begins to enter a spontaneous abreaction or age-regression, it can be helpful for the therapist to avoid pursuing the affects and to focus more on a distanced, cognitive view of the events. For example, in an MPD patient, if a terrified child alter emerges, it might be helpful first to engage briefly with this alter and then to talk over to ask for more adult observers or helpers. They may be asked to comment on what is occurring and whether the "whole mind" is committed to working on the current flashback at this time for the purpose of healing and mastery. Early in treatment, the answer is usually negative. In a dissociative patient without MPD, the therapist can observe that it seems premature to work on this memory and to ask the patient to move to a more self-observing, adult mode to understand better the work that needs to be done.

Hypnotic distancing techniques with or without the induction of formal trance can be very helpful in this patient population (Fine 1991; Hammond 1990; Kluft 1989; Putnam 1989; Spiegel 1989). Early in treatment it is helpful to teach the patient hypnotic techniques for symptom control. Frequently all that is necessary is to shape self-hypnotic techniques that the patient has already developed. Often, it is empowering for the highly dissociative survivor to realize that he or she is already hypnotically adept and simply needs some expert "coaching" to use hypnotic talents more successfully.

For example, these patients often have an inner "safe place" where they may "go" to achieve peace and calm. The therapist may help patients to learn a brief trance induction to make this process easier and more effective. MPD patients may have a few alters with safe places, but others "don't know" that they could have one too. The therapist may facilitate this with a hypnotic intervention. Hypnotic sleep and/or hypnotic time distortion may be added to increase the efficacy of the safe place image (Kluft 1989).

Another helpful technique is a hypnotic "screen" in the mind on which imagery can be projected. Disturbing visual imagery can be placed on the screen with an attenuation of affect (Spiegel 1989). A hypnotic remote control with on-off, fast forward, reverse, freeze frame, slow motion, image-size reduction, split-screen, zoom in, zoom out, and other features may be very effective in permitting the survivor a greater sense of control over working with traumatic memories. The therapist may work to help the patient learn to bring a disturbing traumatic image voluntarily onto the hypnotic screen to learn how to "turn it off" or to modulate it with the hypnotic remote control. Dissociative survivors are often very skeptical of this approach because so much of their energy is absorbed in attempting to suppress and avoid these intrusive images. However, the survivor's success at doing this voluntarily can be an important step in gaining some sense of mastery and control over PTSD symptoms. Survivors who have been filmed while being abused or who report a history of involvement in child pornography may find this technique too triggering, however. Reading a hypnotic book about the experience or simply describing someone else having it may be a useful substitute for the screen image in these and other patients (Hammond 1990; Kluft 1989).

Other hypnotic techniques to modulate affect include imagery to "turn down" anxiety, such as an internal rheostat or control system; a hypnotic time vault where traumatic memories can be placed until they can be worked on again; and various imagery techniques to help the patient with anger, feelings of vulnerability, and the burdens of the past. Techniques that tend to increase affect, such as hypnotic age-regression and affect bridge, may also be used to increase the intensity of affects when this is therapeutically indicated (Fine 1991; Hammond 1990; Kluft 1989; Putnam 1989; Spiegel 1989). However, it is usually best to postpone use of techniques that intensify affect until the patient has considerable mastery over attenuation of affects by using distancing and pacing techniques.

In many patients, it may become possible to use hypnotic techniques to "fractionate" abreactions (Fine 1991; Kluft 1991). Here, the patient and therapist first achieve a working overview of the patient's history by using distancing techniques. Next, the patient is invited to select some "fraction" or percentage of the total affect of a particular traumatic memory to abreact. It is often possible to schedule such abreactive work for a specific session. Sometimes, scheduling an extended session may be helpful in working on complex traumatic material requiring abreaction. If the patient has MPD, all alters relevant to the particular memory may be invited while others listen in. Supportive hypnotic techniques such as hypnotic time distortion may be used to modulate the intensity of affect during the abreaction and to close down the abreaction before the end of the session to permit the patient to regroup, process the session, and return to his or her usual activities (Steele and Colrain 1990).

It is also important to recognize common fantasies about working with trauma found among dissociative patients. These beliefs and assumptions often have powerful effects on the patient's ability to resolve dissociative symptoms fully (Fine 1991). For example, early in therapy, many dissociative patients insist that rapid, intense derepression of traumatic memories—"letting it all hang out"—will achieve recovery. This notion often conceals denial of the actual work that must be done to face the meaning of the abuse for the lives of these patients. Dissociative patients often have to face not only the abuse memories but also the implications of these for their whole lives and in their family relationships. Many dissociative patients confront extraordinary pain and grief as they realize the real meaning of family abusiveness. As one MPD patient stated as she achieved a final fusion of all of her alters and became more fully in touch with the meaning of her childhood experiences: "I realize now that I am an orphan, even though my family is still alive."

Many therapists too easily collude with dissociative patients and prematurely enter into intensive abreactive work without adequate stabilization and preparation (Fine 1991; Steele and Colrain 1990). The results are usually disastrous. This approach generally results in a flooded, overwhelmed patient who is now phobic of therapy and less able to use structuring of the dissociative experiences for recovery without additional intensive therapy.

Working-Through of Traumatic Memories

Abreactive work alone is usually insufficient to bring about resolution of a dissociative disorder and unification of the patient's divided mental processes. It is necessary to not only work on the dissociated memories and affects but also on the assumptive world and unconscious fantasies of the dissociative incest survivor (Fine 1990, 1991; Marmer 1991).

The distorted belief system of the dissociative incest survivor often resembles the doublethink propaganda of the totalitarian state in Orwell's *1984* (1949). It may include the following notions (among many others):

1. You must be dissociative (multiple) to be safe.
2. Abuse is inevitable; you can only attempt to make it more predictable and controllable.
3. Physical and sexual abuse itself is not so bad, because the actual experiences can be dissociated. The worst thing is the uncertainty of not knowing when the abuse will occur and having no ability to control it.
4. Love and sex are the same.
5. Anger and violence are the same.
6. Self-destructiveness is safety.
7. All relationships are abusive. You are either a victim or an abuser.
8. Nothing can ever change.
9. There is no freedom to choose anything.

Fine (1988, 1990, 1991) has reviewed in depth the cognitive sequelae of incest and therapeutic approaches to cognitive distortions in the dissociative incest survivor. She suggests a method of treatment that involves inviting the incest survivor to consider alternative hypotheses to his or her beliefs as well as the data that support the belief. Ultimately, using this method, core aspects of the patient's cognitive distortions are systematically confronted.

Marmer (1991) and Spiegel (1991b) both discuss other aspects of working-through of traumatic memories in the dissociative patient. They emphasize the importance of the patient's disclosing without punishment previously secret, forbidden material. The presence of a "witness" to the patient's shame, guilt, and horror are important. Both authors also emphasize the importance of reworking the past to transform the meaning of the unchangeable events and the patient's role in them.

Ultimately, the therapeutic process leads to an integration (Kluft 1986, 1991) or congruence (Spiegel 1991b) between the previously dissociated memories, thoughts, feelings, and assumptions. In MPD patients, this may involve the coalescence of the alters in a "fusion" (Kluft 1986, 1991). In both the MPD patient and the non-MPD dissociative patient, therapy helps develop the capacity to have freely available in consciousness material that was previously maintained by dissociative compartmentalization (Spiegel 1991b).

After dissociative defenses and structures are relinquished, the patient will need additional therapy to learn to live in a nondissociative manner. Also, many patients must rework the therapy material from a unified frame of reference. This may lead to a deepening in understanding as well as an augmentation in pain. The patient can no longer use dissociative "magic" to attenuate the full impact of the life history. Grief work is common during this phase of treatment. Here the patient commonly focuses on the lost years of his or her life, the inability to maintain unrealistic views of family members or others who have mistreated the patient, and the relinquishing of dissociative methods for handling all aspects of life.

Conclusion

Dissociative disorders are common among survivors of incest. Successful treatment of dissociation is possible. However, the clinician must be educated about posttraumatic and dissociative symptoms and psychodynamics in order to work effectively with these patients. Although many dissociative patients require long-term psychotherapy, the outcome may be quite favorable (even if conducted by therapists who are relatively inexperienced in this area) if the treatment is conceptualized and structured properly (Coons 1986). These patients are often rewarding to treat as well. They allow us to see the ability of human beings to survive horrific childhood trauma and to maintain the capacity for warmth, humor, joy, creativity, and caring for others despite abuse.

References

American Psychiatric Association: Diagnostic and Statistical Manual of Mental Disorders, 3rd Edition, Revised. Washington, DC, American Psychiatric Association, 1987

Armstrong JG: The psychological organization of multiple personality disordered patients as revealed in psychological testing. Psychiatr Clin North Am 14:513–516, 1991

Armstrong JG, Loewenstein RJ: Characteristics of patients with multiple personality and dissociative disorders on psychological testing. J Nerv Ment Dis 178:448–454, 1990

Braun BG (ed): The Treatment of Multiple Personality Disorder. Washington, DC, American Psychiatric Press, 1986

Braun BG, Sachs RG: The development of multiple personality disorder: predisposing, precipitating, and perpetuating factors, in Childhood Antecedents of Multiple Personality. Edited by Kluft RP. Washington, DC, American Psychiatric Press, 1985, pp 37–64

Briere J: Therapy for Adults Molested as Children: Beyond Survival. New York, Springer, 1989

Briere J, Conte J: Amnesia in adults molested as children: testing theories of repression. Paper presented at the annual meeting of the American Psychological Association, New Orleans, LA, August 1989

Coons PM: Treatment progress in 20 patients with multiple personality disorder. J Nerv Ment Dis 174:715–721, 1986

Fine CG: Thoughts on the cognitive perceptual substrates of multiple personality disorder. Dissociation 1(4):5–9, 1988

Fine CG: The cognitive sequelae of incest, in Incest-Related Disorders of Adult Psychopathology. Edited by Kluft RP. Washington, DC, American Psychiatric Press, 1990, pp 161–182

Fine CG: Treatment stabilization and crisis prevention: pacing the therapy of the MPD patient. Psychiatr Clin North Am 14:661–675, 1991

Gelinas DJ: The persistent negative effects of incest. Psychiatry 46:312–332, 1983

Goodwin J: Sexual Abuse: Incest Victims and Their Families, 2nd Edition. Chicago, IL, Year Book Medical Publishers, 1989

Hammond DC: Handbook of Hypnotic Suggestions and Metaphors. New York, WW Norton, 1990

Herman JL: Father-Daughter Incest. Cambridge, MA, Harvard University Press, 1981

Kluft RP: Aspects of the treatment of multiple personality disorder. Psychiatric Annals 14:51–55, 1984a

Kluft RP: Treatment of multiple personality disorder. Psychiatr Clin North Am 7:9–29, 1984b

Kluft RP: The treatment of multiple personality disorder (MPD): current concepts, in Directions in Psychiatry. Edited by Flach FF. New York, Hatherleigh, 1985, pp 1–10

Kluft RP: Personality unification in multiple personality disorder: a follow-up study, in Treatment of Multiple Personality Disorder. Edited by Braun BG. Washington, DC, American Psychiatric Press, 1986, pp 29–60

Kluft RP: The dissociative disorders, in The American Psychiatric Press Textbook of Psychiatry. Edited by Talbot JA, Hales RE, Yudofsky SC. Washington, DC, American Psychiatric Press, 1988, pp 557–584

Kluft RP: Playing for time: temporizing techniques in the treatment of multiple personality disorder. Am J Clin Hypn 32:90–97, 1989

Kluft RP: Multiple personality disorder, in American Psychiatric Press Annual Review of Psychiatry, Vol 10. Edited by Tasman A, Goldfinger S. Washington, DC, American Psychiatric Press, 1991, pp 161–188

Kluft RP: Discussion: a specialist's perspective on multiple personality disorder. Psychoanalytic Inquiry 12:139–171, 1992

Lindy JD: Vietnam: A Casebook. New York, Brunner/Mazel, 1988

Loewenstein RJ: Psychogenic amnesia and psychogenic fugue: a comprehensive review, in American Psychiatric Press Review of Psychiatry, Vol 10. Edited by Tasman A, Goldfinger SM. Washington, DC, American Psychiatric Press, 1991a, pp 189–222

Loewenstein RJ: An office mental status examination for chronic complex dissociative symptoms and multiple personality disorder. Psychiatr Clin North Am 14:567–604, 1991b

Loewenstein RJ: Posttraumatic and dissociative aspects of transference and countertransference in the treatment of multiple personality disorder, in Clinical Perspectives on Multiple Personality Disorder. Edited by Kluft RP, Fine CG. Washington, DC, American Psychiatric Press (in press)

Loewenstein RJ, Putnam FW: The clinical phenomenology of males with multiple personality disorder. Dissociation 3:135–143, 1990

Loewenstein RJ, Ross D: Multiple personality and psychoanalysis: an introduction. Psychoanalytic Inquiry 12:3–48, 1992

Loewenstein RJ, Hornstein N, Farber B: Open trial of clonazepam in the treatment of posttraumatic stress symptoms in MPD. Dissociation 1(3):3–12, 1988

Ludwig AM: The psychobiological functions of dissociation. Am J Clin Hypn 26:93–99, 1983

Marmer S: Multiple personality disorder: a psychoanalytic perspective. Psychiatr Clin North Am 14:677–693, 1991

Orwell G: Nineteen Eighty-Four. New York, Harcourt Brace, 1949

Peebles-Kleiger MJ: Using countertransference in the hypnosis of trauma victims: a model for turning hazard into healing. Am J Psychother 43:518–530, 1989

Putnam FW: Dissociation as a response to extreme trauma, in Childhood Antecedents of Multiple Personality. Edited by Kluft RP. Washington, DC, American Psychiatric Press, 1985, pp 65–97

Putnam FW: Diagnosis and Treatment of Multiple Personality Disorder. New York, Guilford, 1989

Putnam FW: Dissociative phenomena, in American Psychiatric Press Review of Psychiatry, Vol 10. Edited by Tasman A, Goldfinger SM. Washington, DC, American Psychiatric Press, 1991, pp 145–160

Ross CA: The epidemiology of multiple personality disorder and dissociation. Psychiatr Clin North Am 14:503–517, 1991

Ross CA: Multiple Personality Disorder: Diagnosis, Clinical Features, and Treatment. New York, Wiley, 1989

Ross CA, Joshi S, Currie R: Dissociative experiences in the general population. Am J Psychiatry 147:1547–1552, 1990

Spiegel D: Dissociation, double binds, and posttraumatic stress, in The Treatment of Multiple Personality Disorder. Edited by Braun BG. Washington, DC, American Psychiatric Association, 1986, pp 61–77

Spiegel D: Dissociation and hypnosis in posttraumatic stress disorders. Journal of Traumatic Stress Studies 1:17–33, 1988

Spiegel D: Hypnosis in the treatment of victims of sexual abuse. Psychiatr Clin North Am 12:295–305, 1989

Spiegel D: Trauma, dissociation, and hypnosis, in Incest-Related Disorders of Adult Psychopathology. Edited by Kluft RP. Washington, DC, American Psychiatric Press, 1990, pp 247–261

Spiegel D: Dissociation and trauma, in American Psychiatric Press Review of Psychiatry, Vol 10. Edited by Tasman A, Goldfinger SM. Washington, DC, American Psychiatric Press, 1991a, pp 261–275

Spiegel D: The dissociative disorders, in American Psychiatric Press Review of Psychiatry, Vol 10. Edited by Tasman A, Goldfinger SM. Washington, DC, American Psychiatric Press, 1991b, pp 141–276

Steele K, Colrain J: Abreactive work with sexual abuse survivors: concepts and techniques, in The Sexually Abused Male, Vol 2. Edited by Hunter M. Lexington, MA, Lexington Books, 1990, pp 1–55

Turkus J: Psychotherapy and case management for multiple personality disorder: synthesis for continuity of care. Psychiatr Clin North Am 14:649–660, 1991

van der Kolk B: Psychological Trauma. Washington, DC, American Psychiatric Press, 1986

Chapter 5

The Role of Medications in Treating Adult Survivors of Childhood Trauma

José A. Saporta, Jr., M.D.
J. Case, M.D.

*T*his chapter will discuss the role of psychopharmacology in the treatment of adults who are experiencing the effects of childhood trauma. We will present a rationale for the use of medications for these patients, including ameliorating posttraumatic symptoms that impair the patient's ability to utilize psychotherapy and improving quality of life by relieving other posttraumatic symptoms and treating coexisting syndromes. We will apply and extend the current biological model for posttraumatic stress disorder (PTSD) in order to understand how various medications might work. We speculate that medications restore the patient's capacity to modulate certain basic neurobiologic functions that are disrupted by overwhelming stress. We will then discuss those medications used to treat PTSD symptoms and other symptoms that are common among adult victims of child abuse. Finally, we will present and discuss special problems frequently encountered when one integrates pharmacotherapy into the psychotherapy of adults who were traumatized as children.

Existing Sources of Information

Given the paucity of research in this area, we are left to draw on other sources for guiding a pharmacologic approach to the adult child abuse

---

It would be impossible to acknowledge each instance in which our ideas in this chapter were influenced by our teacher, colleague, and friend Bessel A. van der Kolk, M.D. We also thank Anne Ling Li, M.D., for her editorial expertise.

survivor. A PTSD model has been useful in understanding many of these patients (Coons et al. 1989, 1990; Goodwin 1985), and we may look to the literature on the pharmacotherapy of PTSD for help (Davidson et al. 1990; Friedman 1988; van der Kolk 1987). While useful, this literature is limited for several reasons. First, there is little known about the pharmacotherapy of PTSD as such, with too few controlled trials beginning as recently as 1988. Furthermore, those medications that have been studied have been moderately effective at best. Second, the subjects studied have predominantly been male combat veterans who were traumatized as adults. It is not clear how generalizable these findings are to a population that is mostly women who have been traumatized earlier in life and often throughout childhood, and who have been exposed to other pathogenic influences in their childhood environment. Finally, although many of these patients clearly have PTSD, others may not, and still others may have complex and atypical forms of PTSD. We need studies of adult survivors of child abuse as such to better inform our treatment.

Another source of help is the limited literature on the pharmacotherapy of borderline personality disorder (BPD; Cowdry and Gardner 1988; Gardner and Cowdry 1989; Soloff 1989). Although these studies do not address the etiologic role of trauma in these patients, recent research would suggest that many of these subjects have histories of childhood trauma (Brown and Anderson 1991; Herman et al. 1989; Ogata et al. 1990). Thus, medications found helpful for subjects in these studies may be applicable to the population that we are considering. However, we do not know whether the presence of childhood trauma or PTSD symptoms mitigate drug response in borderline patients. We also do not know if findings from these studies are applicable to nonborderline patients who share symptoms that were targeted by these studies. Although these studies may suggest medications for empirical trials, the complicating factors mentioned cry out for further study.

Third, these patients frequently suffer from other Axis I psychiatric syndromes, which will be discussed later in this chapter. In these cases, we recommend a standard approach to these syndromes as suggested by the existing literature. Furthermore, certain atypical syndromes may have a specific pharmacologic response, such as the response of atypical depression/hysteroid dysphoria to monoamine oxidase inhibitors (MAOIs; Liebowitz et al. 1988; Quitkin et al. 1989) or the response of "unstable" or "impulsive" character disorders to lithium (Rifkin et al.

1972; Sheard 1971; Wickman and Reed 1987). Traumatized patients may show similar problems and perhaps a similar pharmacologic response.

Finally, our discussion is informed by our clinical experience. We have treated many of these patients in outpatient pharmacotherapy as well as through our function as psychiatrists on an inpatient unit specializing in treatment of adults who have been traumatized as children. We are eager to see our anecdotal experience either supported or refuted by future research.

Indications for Pharmacotherapy in Posttraumatic Patients

There are several indications for medications in adults who have been abused as children:

1. Posttraumatic symptoms may specifically impair the patient's ability to utilize psychotherapy. These symptoms are based in abnormal or excessive physiologic responses and are often responsive to medications.
2. Pharmacologic intervention aimed at controlling bodily based PTSD symptoms can improve the patient's comfort and quality of life outside of therapy as well. This may be a sufficient reason for medical intervention, which, in turn, may enhance psychological recovery.
3. The patient's quality of life and ability to utilize psychotherapy may be impaired by other psychiatric syndromes that may be pharmacologically responsive.

Medication and Psychotherapy

Psychotherapy is an essential component in the treatment of posttraumatic reactions. However, many posttraumatic symptoms specifically impair the patient's capacity to engage in psychotherapy. Many of these symptoms are most likely based in trauma-induced neurobiologic changes. Let us look more specifically at various ways in which PTSD symptoms can interfere with psychotherapy.

1. Traumatized patients may be conditioned to react to reminders of the traumatic event, as well as to other contemporary stresses with

overwhelming physiologic emergency responses (Blanchard et al. 1982; McFall et al. 1990; Pitman et al. 1987). This contributes to "all-or-none" emotional reactions. Thus, whenever the therapeutic work touches on any reminders of the trauma (and in some cases whenever any emotionally charged material is brought forth), this triggers a terrifying physiological and emotional response. As a result, these patients do not feel safe in their own bodies; thus, they are unable to feel sufficiently safe in the therapeutic relationship to explore and integrate frightening and painful memories.

2. Overwhelming trauma shatters the victim's sense of control over his or her life and may establish an external locus of control. When therapy repeatedly triggers bodily reactions that are out of the patient's control, then therapy may perpetuate a sense of loss of control, helplessness, and external locus of control. This further undermines the individual's competence and subverts the therapeutic goal of empowering the patient.

3. Baseline high levels of autonomic arousal and anxiety interfere with cognition. In severe cases, there may be gross disorganization of thinking in extreme states of arousal. Extreme arousal, then, impairs the patient's ability to put feelings and memories into perspective and to learn new coping strategies.

4. Finally, the emotional and cognitive constriction seen in PTSD cuts off the individual's access to an inner world of fantasy and symbols (van der Kolk 1987). In severe cases, tension and affects may be discharged directly into action without intervening thought. Thus, the individual's capacity to put his or her experience into words as well as to find new meanings is compromised.

Medications can thus enhance psychotherapy by decreasing overwhelming bodily reactions and restoring the patient's control over these bodily responses. The patient's experience of safety is thereby increased, which is essential for psychotherapy. Medications should decrease the baseline level of arousal and thereby improve cognitive function. They may also allow the individual greater access to an inner world of fantasy and symbols and interpose thought between impulse and action. Uncontrolled physiologic reactions undermine the patient's emotional well-being and sense of competence in his or her life outside of therapy as well. Coexisting psychiatric syndromes can further impair the patient's comfort and ability to function. The goal of pharmacotherapy, then, is to improve the patient's capacity to utilize psychotherapy and to improve functioning and reduce suffering in other areas of life.

Target Symptoms for Pharmacotherapy

PTSD Symptoms

Effective pharmacotherapy of trauma-related syndromes requires careful identification and monitoring of target symptoms. The type of medication indicated is determined by the most prominent target symptoms and may vary from patient to patient. Target symptoms can be categorized as

1. Core PTSD symptoms;
2. Symptoms seen frequently in PTSD and other posttraumatic states but not essential to the diagnosis; and
3. Symptoms of common comorbid conditions such as various forms of depression, eating disorders, dissociative disorders, and so on.

Core PTSD symptoms can be divided into "positive" and "negative" symptom clusters (intrusive versus avoidance symptom clusters; Horowitz 1986). This is analogous to the distinction between positive and negative symptoms in schizophrenia. Positive symptoms consist of autonomic hyperarousal and hyperreactivity, and reexperiencing phenomena. Autonomic arousal manifests as persistent anxiety and tension, insomnia, hyperactive startle reactions, and physiologic reactivity upon exposure to events reminiscent of or associated with the original traumas. Reexperiencing can take the form of flashbacks, nightmares, and motoric reenactments. These experiences are often preceded by or occur in the context of physiologic arousal (Rainey et al. 1987). Traumatic memories may be stored in fragmented form and may intrude into consciousness in the form of visual images, auditory hallucinations usually heard inside the head, as well as various somatic sensations and hallucinations in any sensory modality. Panic and rage attacks also occur. Irritable outbursts along with an overall inability to modulate aggression are frequent. Aggression is often turned against the self in various forms of self-abuse and self-mutilation.

Negative symptoms consist of emotional numbing and cognitive constriction, which may lead to anhedonia, social withdrawal, and decreased occupational functioning. Experience and research suggest that the positive symptoms of PTSD are more medication-responsive, whereas the negative symptoms can be resistant to medical treatment. Interestingly, although positive PTSD symptoms may also respond to behavioral or implosive therapy, negative or avoidant PTSD symptoms appear to be resistant to this form of treatment as well (Keane et al., in press).

Many symptoms of BPD overlap with PTSD symptoms (Herman and van der Kolk 1987), such as impulsivity, affective instability, and poorly modulated aggression. Furthermore, the two syndromes may interact. For example, self-mutilation or aggressive outbursts often occur during states of overwhelming arousal. Affect intolerance and primitive defenses may be exacerbated by conditioned physiologic emergency responses. In these cases, pharmacologic focus on PTSD symptoms, such as improving the patient's capacity to modulate arousal, may help to stabilize dysfunction secondary to character pathology.

Other Psychiatric Syndromes

Adult survivors of child abuse are vulnerable to a number of other psychiatric difficulties that may require pharmacologic intervention. Some of the more frequently encountered syndromes in our experience include the following.

Affective disorders.   Depression is extremely common in this population (Schetky 1990). Patients can present with major depressive episodes, dysthymia, and atypical depressions. Depression in the context of PTSD among war veterans is regarded as psychologically and biologically distinct from major depression occurring without PTSD and is more resistant to standard antidepressant agents (Southwick et al. 1991). This is probably also true for PTSD that is secondary to child abuse. Bipolar and cyclothymic conditions are also seen and are discussed in a later section.

Anxiety disorders.   Traumatized patients may present with various anxiety symptoms in addition to PTSD. They may experience generalized anxiety, panic attacks with or without agoraphobia, and various phobias. Anxiety attacks may occur as part of a flashback experience; these are distinguished from panic attacks in that the former are in response to meaningful stimuli associated with the trauma. Phobias may be related to traumatic associations. We have also seen patients present with seemingly autonomous panic attacks, to be followed in due course by recollections of childhood abuse and the onset of PTSD symptoms. We do not know if these are coincidental occurrences or if they are psychophysiologically related. Panic attacks and other anxiety symptoms in childhood trauma survivors tend to respond to similar pharmacologic interventions, including clonazepam, tricyclic antidepressants (TCAs), MAOIs, and fluoxetine.

Eating disorders. These disorders, including anorexia, bulimia, and mixed conditions, are frequently associated with histories of sexual or physical abuse (Damlouji and Ferguson 1985; Demitrack et al. 1990; Goldfarb 1987). Eating disorders can complicate the pharmacologic management of other symptoms, as certain medications are associated with weight gain (lithium, TCAs, MAOIs).

Substance abuse disorders. These are quite frequent concomitants of PTSD, or they may appear with other syndromes among child abuse survivors. Often these patients have been using substances in order to treat symptoms of PTSD. In these cases, more specific management of PTSD symptoms with standard drugs may help prevent relapse. Some patients are resistant to using medications after they have achieved sobriety. Psychoeducation and patient collaboration are necessary before such patients will agree to a trial of medications.

Dissociative disorders. These disorders, including psychogenic amnesia and fugue, depersonalization disorder, multiple personality disorder (MPD), and dissociative disorder not otherwise specified (DDNOS), are not uncommon as a consequence of childhood trauma. They are discussed elsewhere in this book. Medications play a limited role in managing these conditions, which will be discussed later in this chapter.

Character dysfunction and character disorders. These disorders are commonly seen in child abuse survivors. BPD is particularly relevant here, and its overlap and interaction with PTSD symptoms are discussed in a previous section. Medication management of personality disorders, like the pharmacotherapy of PTSD, requires a specific focus on target symptoms. These symptoms may be PTSD symptoms or other comorbid symptoms discussed throughout this chapter.

In general, clinicians should manage symptoms coexisting with PTSD in the same way as they manage these syndromes when not complicated by PTSD. Thus, major depression is treated with antidepressants; bulimia is treated with fluoxetine or other antidepressants (Enas et al. 1989; Walsh et al. 1991). However, we offer the following caveats. First, traumatized patients may be exquisitely sensitive to medication side effects. This may be a function of the adrenergic hypersensitivity inherent to PTSD, as well as a consequence of the patient's hypervigilance. Posttraumatic hypervigilance often includes an increased focus upon and fear of physical changes and subjective experiences. These patients often need detailed accounts of side effects they might possibly experience and may need reassurance and support when experiencing side effects. Lower starting doses with slower increases may avoid these problems. Second, it may be useful to select an agent that addresses both the salient PTSD symptoms as well as the troubling coexisting symptom. Third, there are medications whose effects may exacerbate symptoms of PTSD. For example, adrenergically stimulating agents, such as desipramine and protriptyline for depression, or stimulants, such as methylphenidate for dysthymia, could potentially worsen symptoms of hyperarousal.

The Psychobiology of Trauma

This section will present a biological model for PTSD and the neurobiological abnormalities thought to underlie posttraumatic symptoms.

Catecholamines and Inescapable Stress

Stress-induced abnormalities in catecholamine regulation and, in particular, the noradrenergic system have been most implicated as the neurobiological underpinning for PTSD symptoms. Bessel van der Kolk and others have proposed the model of inescapable shock in animals as a psychological and biological model for PTSD in humans (Kolb 1987; Krystal et al. 1989; van der Kolk et al. 1985). The biological effects of inescapable stress (IS) in animals may also explain how medications might work to ameliorate PTSD symptoms.

IS in animals produces a syndrome of profound behavioral deficits known as learned helplessness (Maier and Seligman 1976), which parallels the negative symptoms or avoidance phase of PTSD (van der Kolk et al. 1985). Animals exposed to IS are also hyperreactive to subsequent stress, in a manner similar to PTSD patients.

Biochemically, IS produces a massive overutilization of catecholamines, leading to a net depletion of brain catecholamine levels (Anisman et al. 1981; Sherman and Petty 1980; Weiss et al. 1975). Catecholamine overutilization followed by depletion becomes a conditioned response to subsequent mild stress (Anisman and Sklar 1979) as well as a response to contextual cues associated with the inescapable stress (Cassens et al. 1980). This model suggests that humans with PTSD are conditioned to respond to stress with repeated, transient catecholamine overutilization, followed by net depletion of catecholamine stores. The negative or avoidance symptoms of PTSD are thus attributed to catecholamine depletion, whereas hyperactive catecholamine responses are thought to underlie hyperarousal and other "positive" PTSD symptoms.

The hyperactive catecholamine response—and by inference, hyperarousal and overreactivity to stress—may have two mechanisms. First, there is dysregulation of the locus coeruleus. The locus coeruleus is the source of most of the brain's noradrenaline and mediates fear and alarm reactions, or the "trauma response" (Krystal et al. 1989). Drugs that inhibit the locus coeruleus will prevent or ameliorate the effects of IS, whereas drugs that stimulate the locus coeruleus will exacerbate the behavioral and biochemical response to IS. Van der Kolk and others (Krystal et al. 1989; van der Kolk et al. 1985) have suggested that hyperarousal, autonomic hyperreactivity, and increased startle are due to hyperreactivity at the level of the locus coeruleus. Nightmares and flashbacks may be related to hyperpotentiation of neural tracts from the locus coeruleus to the limbic system and may account for the vivid quality of these experiences (van der Kolk et al. 1985).

Another mechanism for excessive noradrenergic responses may be hypersensitivity, or up-regulation of adrenergic postsynaptic receptors (van der Kolk et al. 1985). This may occur in response to the repeated catecholamine depletion discussed previously. Thus, small amounts of catecholamines may elicit an excessive physiologic response.

Physiologic research of PTSD patients supports the analogy between the biology of IS in animals and the human trauma response.

Numerous studies have documented conditioned autonomic reactivity to stimuli reminiscent of the original trauma as measured by heart rate, blood pressure, electromyogram (EMG), and electroencephalogram (EEG) evoked potentials (Blanchard et al. 1982; Dobbs and Wilson 1960; McFall et al. 1990; Paige et al. 1990; Pitman et al. 1987, 1990a). Biochemical studies have also confirmed excessive adrenergic activity in the form of increased 24-hour catecholamines in plasma and urine (Kosten et al. 1987) and receptor changes consistent with exposure to elevated levels of circulating catecholamines (Lerer et al. 1987b; Perry et al. 1987). It is not clear whether these findings represent baseline elevations of norepinephrine or whether they measure phasic elevations of catecholamines superimposed on baseline normal or even depleted catecholamine levels. In further support of the IS model for PTSD, it is those medications that prevent or reverse the effects of IS in animals that have been found useful in reducing PTSD symptoms.

It is not clear how applicable this model of adrenergic reactivity is for child abuse survivors. When adult child abuse survivors meet diagnostic criteria for PTSD, we suspect that the model applies as much to them as to combat survivors. Furthermore, patients with BPD show adrenergic receptor changes similar to those seen in combat veterans with PTSD (Southwick et al. 1990).

Serotonin

We believe that serotonin dysfunction also plays a role in PTSD symptoms. First, there is evidence that severe stress can deplete serotonin levels in animals (Hodge and Butcher 1974; Sherman and Petty 1980; Valzelli 1969, 1982; Valzelli and Bernasconi 1979; Welch and Welch 1971). Desipramine may reverse the effects of inescapable stress in rodents by increasing serotonin in the septum (Sherman and Petty 1980), and pure serotonin agonists will also reverse the effects of inescapable stress (Giral et al. 1988). Second, serotonin systems appear to modulate noradrenergic responsiveness and arousal (Depue and Spoont 1986; Gerson and Baldessarini 1980; Samanin and Garattini 1976). Depletion of serotonin in animals leads to hyperarousal, increased reactivity, increased aggression, and increased response to amphetamines (Breese et al. 1974; Davis and Sheard 1976; Depue and Spoont 1986; Gerson and Baldessarini 1980; Poschlova et al. 1977; Samanin and Garattini 1976). Thus, serotonin abnormalities may con-

tribute to the noradrenergic dysregulation seen in PTSD. Third, serotonin dysfunction may also underlie the proclivity to explosive and
impulsive rage reactions seen in traumatized patients. Depue and
Spoont (1986) characterize the phenomena produced in animals by
serotonin depletion as hyperirritability, hyperexcitability, and hypersensitivity, and an "exaggerated emotional arousal and/or aggressive
display (though not necessarily attack) to relatively mild stimuli . . . "
(p. 55). This description bears a striking resemblance to the phenomenology of PTSD.

Decreased serotonin function has been correlated with hostility,
impulsivity, and self-directed aggression in patients with depression
and with personality disorders, including BPD (Asberg et al. 1976;
Brown et al. 1979; Coccaro et al. 1989). Low-serotonin-mediated
impulsive aggression seems to be a trait that cuts across diagnostic
groups (van Kammen 1987). The research papers discussing low serotonin levels in these patients seem to assume that they are dealing with
a genetic trait. However, other studies of patients with these problems
consistently demonstrate histories of childhood abuse and neglect
(Green 1978; Pattison and Kahan 1983). It is reasonable to suppose that
in child abuse survivors who have difficulties with impulsivity and
self-directed aggression, these problems have been caused by a combination of environmental stress and genetic vulnerability, leading to
decreased serotonin function.

It appears that serotonin mediates a behavioral inhibition system in
the brain (Depue and Spoont 1986; Gray 1987; Soubrié 1986). Behaviors that are motivated by emergency responses or by previous reward
may need to be suppressed if circumstances change. For example, when
previously rewarded behaviors are now punished, or when one per-
ceives a mismatch between the expected outcome of a behavioral
response and the actual, current outcome, then ongoing behaviors are
suppressed. This suppression of behavioral responses depends upon the
behavioral inhibition system that is mediated by serotonin. Drugs that
deplete serotonin thus disinhibit behaviors that would ordinarily be
suppressed. Saporta and van der Kolk have argued elsewhere that
stress-induced serotonin dysfunction may lead to impaired function of
the behavioral inhibition system, which may then underlie various
behavioral problems seen in PTSD, including impulsivity, aggressive
outbursts, compulsive reenactment of trauma-related behavior patterns,
and a seeming inability to learn from past mistakes (Saporta and van

der Kolk, in press; van der Kolk and Saporta, in press).

Finally, serotonin dysfunction appears to be related to obsessive-compulsive disorder (Winslow and Insel 1990) and may underlie the obsessive fixation on the trauma and repetitive intrusion of traumatic memories into consciousness. However, all of these speculations await empirical study.

Endogenous Opioids

There is evidence that the emotional numbing seen in PTSD may be due to an abnormal conditioned endogenous opioid response. IS in animals leads to a conditioned stress-induced analgesia, which is mediated by endogenous opioids (Fanselow 1986; Lewis et al. 1980; Maier 1986). Such a stress-induced analgesia has been shown in combat veterans with PTSD by Pitman, van der Kolk, and colleagues (Pitman et al. 1990b; van der Kolk et al. 1989). Self-reports accompanying the analgesic response in these subjects indicated a relative blunting of emotional responses to the traumatic stimulus.

Abnormalities in endogenous opioids have also been linked to self-mutilating behaviors that occur in traumatized persons (Coid et al. 1983). These behaviors have been reported to follow adult trauma in three cases without a prior history of child abuse (Greenspan and Samuel 1989; Pitman 1990). Kosten and Krystal (1988) speculate that opiate abuse in PTSD patients may serve to decrease arousal and self-medicate other PTSD symptoms, by virtue of the fact that opiates inhibit the locus coeruleus. They point to the similarities between the hyperarousal seen in PTSD and that seen in opioid withdrawal states. Van der Kolk (1989) speculates that self-mutilation and compulsive reexposure to traumatic stress in traumatized patients may serve to induce endogenous opioid production in an attempt to decrease hyperarousal and depersonalization. Subjectively, patients report mounting tension, arousal, and dissociation in response to stress, most notably abandonment. They are analgesic for the self-harm, which is followed by a state of calm.

The models discussed here suggest mechanisms by which medication may work to decrease PTSD symptoms. The goal is to decrease noradrenergic responsivity and improve the modulation of arousal. TCAs, MAOIs, benzodiazepines, and clonidine all inhibit the locus coeruleus and may thus decrease arousal, flashbacks, and nightmares via this mechanism. TCAs and MAOIs may also increase central cate-cholamine stores and thus combat learned helplessness and other negative symptoms, such as decreased motivation, social withdrawal, and anhedonia. TCAs and MAOIs may also eventually down-regulate adrenergic postsynaptic receptors (Charney et al. 1981) and may thereby decrease adrenergic reactivity and other positive PTSD symptoms.

Perhaps more true to the neurologic complexity of the phenomena would be a goal of normalizing the interaction of catecholamine and serotonin systems in the brain. Thus, fluoxetine, lithium, and other serotonergic agonists may enhance the ability of serotonin systems to modulate adrenergic responsiveness and arousal. Improved serotonin function may also improve modulation of aggression and decrease impulsivity.

Medications Used for Posttraumatic Symptoms

Unfortunately, the clinical data on the pharmacotherapy of PTSD is not as impressive as the model described previously would suggest. Several reviews of the literature on the pharmacotherapy of PTSD have been published (Davidson et al. 1990; Friedman 1988; van der Kolk 1987). We will briefly refer to this literature and discuss our experience in applying these findings to adult survivors of childhood trauma.

TCAs and MAO Inhibitors

TCAs and MAOIs are those medications most traditionally studied and used for PTSD. Hogben and Cornfield (1981) first reported dramatic responses in an open trial with phenelzine in treating combat veterans with severe and chronic PTSD. A later open trial with Israeli combat veterans and a controlled trial with Israeli combat veterans and civilian trauma survivors failed to replicate this positive experience (Lerer et al. 1987a; Shestatsky et al. 1988). Other uncontrolled studies showed mild to moderate success at best. Hogben and Cornfield (1981) reported that phenelzine stimulated "intense abreactions" in some of their patients, accompanied by rage. Van der Kolk (1983) also noted that phenelzine induced increased vividness of daytime traumatic memories in veterans with PTSD. We have observed this reaction in patients with PTSD secondary to child abuse.

The results with TCAs in open trials have been similarly mixed. There are only three adequately controlled studies to date. Frank and colleagues (1988) studied imipramine and phenelzine. They showed improvement in positive PTSD symptoms but no change in the negative or avoidance symptoms, as well as no change in global measures of anxiety or depression. Reist and colleagues (1989) showed contrary results with desipramine, with no change in either positive or negative PTSD symptoms but some improvement in symptoms of depression. More recently, Davidson and colleagues (1990) studied amitriptyline and showed improvement in depression, anxiety, and both positive and negative PTSD symptoms. Their study is significant in that while their subjects' depressive symptoms responded within 4 weeks, reduction in PTSD symptoms were not evident until after 8 weeks. They suggest that it may take up to several months to fully realize the benefits of TCAs for PTSD symptoms. However, the results of the Davidson study were moderate at best, and the majority of these patients still met symptom criteria for PTSD at the end of the study.

We believe that TCAs and MAOIs are not particularly effective in patients with severe or chronic PTSD. We also infrequently use these agents in patients with PTSD secondary to child abuse. They may be useful for adult trauma survivors who have a straightforward major depression or panic disorder uncomplicated by other PTSD symptoms. They may also be tried if other regimens fail.

Other Medications

Several other medications have been found useful in PTSD, although none have been subjected to adequately controlled study. Clonidine inhibits the locus coeruleus and has been found effective in reducing hyperarousal, flashbacks, and nightmares in veterans with PTSD (Kolb et al. 1984). We have found clonidine occasionally useful in adult survivors of severe child abuse for whom other medications have failed to control overwhelming arousal accompanied by racing thoughts, flashbacks, and intrusive images and thoughts about their traumas. Clonidine has also been occasionally useful in our experience for decreasing self-mutilating impulses, particularly when accompanied by hyperarousal.

Kolb and colleagues (1984) found propranolol helpful for the positive symptoms of PTSD, although less so than clonidine. Propranolol has also been found helpful in children with PTSD (Famularo et al. 1988). In van der Kolk's (1987) experience, management of chronic PTSD symptoms in combat veterans required doses in excess of 600 mg per day, which led to unacceptable side effects.

Carbamazepine has been shown to be effective in two open trials in decreasing hyperarousal, nightmares, and flashbacks (Lipper et al. 1986; Wolf et al. 1988). Carbamazepine also decreases impulsive self-destructive behavior in patients with BPD, according to controlled studies (Cowdry and Gardner 1988; Gardner and Cowdry 1986). Thus, carbamazepine would be a reasonable choice for patients with PTSD symptomatology complicated by impulsivity and self-mutilation.

Most recently, an open trial found that valproic acid decreased symptoms of hyperarousal/hyperreactivity and avoidant/withdrawal symptoms and improved sleep in combat veterans with chronic PTSD (Fesler 1991). There was no effect on reexperiencing symptoms. We find valproic acid occasionally helpful in adult survivors of child abuse whose PTSD is complicated by marked affective instability and impulsive rage reactions.

The finding that both carbamazepine and valproic acid may be useful in reducing PTSD symptoms has suggested another biological model for PTSD based upon the phenomenon of "kindling" (Lipper et al. 1986; van der Kolk 1987; van der Kolk et al. 1985; Wolf et al. 1988). According to this model, repeated stimulation of neural structures causes them and areas adjacent or connected to them to become hypersensitive (Post and Kopanda 1976). Eventually, these structures fire spontaneously and inappropriately without stimulation. Progressively worsening PTSD symptoms may be related to an analogous process occurring in the limbic systems of chronic PTSD patients.

Benzodiazepines are useful in helping patients sleep and in decreasing overwhelmingly strong emotional reactions (van der Kolk 1987). Given the high incidence of substance abuse problems in these patients, these agents must be used cautiously. We have noted particular success with clonazepam, in divided doses from 1–4 mg daily in decreasing arousal, panic reactions, and nightmares and in improving sleep. Loewenstein and colleagues (1988) have conducted an open trial of clonazepam in patients with MPD and found it effective in decreasing PTSD symptoms.

Lithium can be helpful in treating patients with severe PTSD where poor affect modulation, recurrent depression, impulsivity, and explosive rage reactions are common. Van der Kolk (1983) gave lithium in an open trial to veterans with chronic PTSD who had a proclivity to explosive rage reactions. Eight out of 14 patients showed improvement, with an increased sense of control as well as a decrease in positive PTSD symptoms. Lithium has also been found effective in decreasing impulsivity and self-mutilation and improving affect modulation in patients described as "unstable" or "impulse ridden" and in patients with BPD (Links et al. 1990; Rifkin et al. 1972; Sheard 1971; Wickman and Reed 1987).

The role of fluoxetine and other serotonergic agonists in PTSD awaits study. We have found fluoxetine frequently effective in depression complicated by PTSD, as well as in improving modulation of arousal, improving modulation of rage, decreasing impulsivity, and decreasing both positive and negative PTSD symptoms. Trauma victims may be obsessively fixated on the traumatic event and organize their lives around it. We are finding that fluoxetine helps these patients achieve greater mental flexibility and move beyond their fixation on the trauma. The role of fluoxetine in treating patients with BPD is being explored (Cornelius et al. 1990; Norden 1989).

Antipsychotic Medications

Antipsychotic medications are not a first-line approach to the treatment of posttraumatic symptoms. However, their use is indicated in a number of limited situations. These include both primary PTSD symptoms and symptoms of comorbid psychopathology. Primary PTSD symptoms that may require the use of antipsychotics include reexperiencing phenomena, or flashbacks that take the form of hallucinations, delusions, or extreme agitation.

A brief discussion of the relationship of hallucinations and delusions to PTSD flashbacks is in order. By definition, these experiences are psychotic. They are, however, different from psychotic symptoms seen in other disorders by virtue of the fact that they are a reexperiencing of actual events, albeit at times in distorted form. Thus, the hallucinations and delusions seen in flashbacks may be better conceptualized as dissociative phenomena and may be related to psychotic-like symptoms seen in the dissociative disorders. These phenomena may have been what previous clinicians meant by the concept of hysterical psychosis. It is reasonable to suppose that the underlying neurophysiology of these psychotic experiences differs from the hallucinations and delusions seen, for instance, in schizophrenia. This may account for our impression that flashback-related psychotic symptoms respond less well to antipsychotic medications than hallucinations and delusions associated with schizophrenia or affective disorders. However, in severe or chronic cases, where other agents used to decrease flashbacks have failed, even a small chance of benefit may be worth the risk.

Severe flashbacks, then, can include both hallucinatory and delusional experiences. Hallucinations can be in any sensory modality (most often visual, tactile, and auditory) and are an actual reexperiencing of an aspect of the patient's past. Most often, these experiences are brief and the subject can easily be "grounded" (i.e., helped to reality test that these experiences are not happening in the here and now). If these measures are not effective, an oral or intramuscular dose of lorazepam can relieve the individual of the terrifying experience. There are severe cases, however, which can last hours or even days, and patients can be totally out of touch with their environment during this time. In such cases, the judicious use of antipsychotics can (in our experience) help to calm patients and decrease the intensity of these experiences. Often, the effects seem more specific than just due to sedation; patients on neuroleptics experience a diminution of hallucinatory symptoms and an ability to test reality that they did not achieve with benzodiazepines.

Delusional experiences can also accompany flashbacks. For example, the patient may believe that he or she is being abused or in danger of assault by a relative who is now dead. When these thoughts are persistent, not amenable to reality testing, and not eliminated by other agents used to control flashbacks, then low-dose antipsychotics may be helpful.

In extreme cases, periods of intense agitation and even assaultiveness can accompany flashbacks. Acute management of these episodes may require the use of antipsychotics in a manner similar to the management of acute agitation in other psychotic states.

Finally, a patient's persistent and overwhelming anxiety may respond poorly to even high doses of benzodiazepines (e.g., 10 mg of clonazepam per day), and the patient may be unable to tolerate other options, such as clonidine. In these cases, low-dose antipsychotics are a reasonable option.

Psychotic symptoms in traumatized patients are not always or necessarily related to flashbacks. They may represent comorbid symptoms that are primarily psychotic. Such symptoms are not uncommon in this population and require the primary use of an antipsychotic. They include the following:

1. Micropsychotic episodes (including psychotic transferences);
2. Major depression with psychotic features;
3. Persistent psychotic symptoms that meet criteria for psychotic disorder, not otherwise specified (NOS); and
4. Psychotic symptoms that may accompany dissociative disorders (including MPD).

Micropsychotic episodes (MEs) are brief periods of impaired reality testing that are often precipitated by stress. They are not flashbacks in that they are not a reexperiencing of a past event (although the differential diagnosis between MEs and flashback-related psychotic symptoms may be difficult). MEs are seen most frequently in the context of a severe personality disorder. Common presentations in child abuse survivors include periods of paranoid delusions and periods of thought disorder (with ideas of reference and loose associations, with intrusions of primitive material into consciousness being common). Low-dose antipsychotics on an as-needed basis can often relieve these symptoms. If these episodes recur frequently, they can be quite disabling and may call for a standing dose of neuroleptic.

The so-called psychotic transference is a specific type of limited psychotic experience. We have seen a number of cases in which the patient develops a specific delusional response to a clinician (most often a therapist). This is distinct from situations where a clinician triggers anxiety or flashbacks either because of perceived similarities to a past perpetrator of abuse or because of the anticipated exploration or disclosures of memories with this clinician. We are referring instead to a situation in which the patient develops a delusion organized around the therapist. We have found that most such cases do not respond to antipsychotic medication and require transfer of the patient to another therapist or another institution. However, a trial of low-dose neuroleptic should be considered in cases not amenable to other interventions.

Major depressive episodes are common among these patients, and these episodes can be accompanied by psychotic features. In this case, the use of antipsychotics in conjunction with antidepressants in a manner identical to their use in psychotic depression uncomplicated by PTSD is indicated. Psychotic symptoms as part of other psychotic disorders should be managed in a standard fashion.

Patients with MPD often complain of auditory hallucinations (usually heard inside the head) and can experience thought withdrawal, delusions of passive influence, and other symptoms suggestive of schizophrenia (Kluft 1987). However, it is clear that these symptoms rarely respond to antipsychotic medications. They are indicative of a dissociative process that requires psychotherapeutic intervention. Experts in the treatment of MPD argue against the use of neuroleptics in MPD (Loewenstein 1991; Putnam 1989). However, we occasionally encounter cases where hallucinations are very disturbing or dangerous and a careful trial of low-dose neuroleptic medication is helpful. This may be the case for patients with DDNOS, whose voices are dissociative phenomena but do not represent dissociated personality states. Loewenstein (1991) argues that neuroleptics can decrease psychotic and pseudopsychotic symptoms in MPD patients by decreasing anxiety and agitation. However, chronic use of neuroleptics in this population should be avoided as much as possible.

Frequent Problems in Traumatized Patients

Depression

Depression is likely the most common coexisting problem in patients with PTSD and a history of child abuse. Various types of depressive syndromes are commonly seen. We find it useful to diagnose the type of depression independent of the PTSD (i.e., major depression, dysthymia, cyclothymia, rejection-sensitive dysphoria) and then use those agents suggested in the existing literature to be most effective for the category of depression at hand (D. M. Osser, unpublished data, March 1991). The coexistence of PTSD is factored in as a negative prognostic indicator for drug response. In general, we find depression in the context of PTSD in child abuse survivors to be relatively resistant to standard TCAs or MAOIs. Fluoxetine seems promising for the often chronic depression in this population. Some treatment-resistant depressions respond to standard augmentation strategies, such as adding lithium to fluoxetine. We have also seen a number of these depressed patients respond to bupropion, but our experience here is limited.

Patients are frequently depressed during the period of turmoil that accompanies and follows the initial recollection of memories of abuse. We have noted that depression during this period can be resistant to medications. Much of the depression in these patients is overdetermined by shame- and guilt-ridden self-images, chronic helplessness, and rage. Although medication may help alleviate severe depression, patients often need to understand that they must bear some degree of dysphoria and even despair while they work though their difficulties in psychotherapy. In times of despair, they may require reassurance that they will eventually work through these difficulties.

Mood Swings

We often see adult child abuse victims who demonstrate wide fluctuations in mood. Phenomenologically, these patients can appear to be cyclothymic or even to have rapid-cycling bipolar disorder. During periods of elation or agitation, they may engage in impulsive and injudicious behaviors. Their sleep is often disrupted. Hyperaroused patients may report racing thoughts.

Some adult survivors of childhood trauma demonstrate an incapacity to modulate affect, which can lead to marked fluctuations in mood. Physiological and psychological factors contribute to this deficit. Physiologically based difficulties may be due to hyperarousal secondary to PTSD. The inability to modulate arousal and affect may also be traced developmentally to early disruptions in attachments to caretakers, as has been demonstrated in nonhuman primates (Kraemer et al. 1984).

Psychologically, many of these patients show ego deficits in their ability to tolerate affects and in self-soothing. As a result, they are prone to action as a mechanism for managing their dysphoric feelings. Thus, their states of agitation, extreme arousal, fear, and attempts to manage distress through action may be misinterpreted as manic or hypomanic states. These patients may also have contradictory and poorly integrated self-representations, causing them to experience themselves in markedly different ways. Their moods can fluctuate widely with these changes in self-experience. Patients with dissociative psychopathology may experience themselves differently in different dissociative states of mind, leading to dramatic and (at times) rapid mood fluctuations.

The differential diagnosis between mood fluctuations secondary to PTSD and its associated character pathology versus cyclothymia and rapid cycling bipolar illness can be difficult. A family history of bipolar disorder and a past history of clearly delineated depression (including psychotic depression) or mania weight the diagnosis toward a bipolar diathesis. On the other hand, the coexistence of signs and symptoms of hyperarousal, flashbacks, or other PTSD symptoms during supposed hypomanic states, and mood fluctuations in response to meaningful precipitants, may suggest mood fluctuations as secondary to PTSD and associated character pathology. If the patient terminates states of hyperactivity with an act of self-mutilation, then a posttraumatic etiology is likely. Finally, if stereotypic behaviors that can be related to a traumatic experience in the patient's past recur during states of agitation and hyperactivity, then they likely represent a dissociative state.

Obviously, classic bipolar disorder, cyclothymia, and atypical bipolar disorders can coexist with PTSD or dissociative pathology in traumatized patients. Clinical lore suggests that in patients with MPD who also have major depression or bipolar disorder, all of the "alter personalities" will either be depressed or manic during the respective phase of the illness. This postulate requires more rigorous empirical support. We find it occasionally but not always helpful in selecting medications. We have seen patients in whom not all "alter personalities" shared the same predominant mood state, but for whom some form of thymoleptic was indicated and occasionally effective.

When patients are hyperaroused and show other PTSD symptoms associated with mood swings, treating the primary PTSD symptoms with the agents discussed here will often improve affect modulation. We have seen patients respond to fluoxetine with a decrease in arousal and a leveling of mood fluctuations. Where there seems to be a fundamental problem in modulating affect, lithium can be effective, as we have discussed. We often combine lithium with fluoxetine or clonazepam in managing mood instability and PTSD. At times, we have turned to carbamazepine or valproic acid in managing extreme or rapid fluctuations in mood. In these cases, the distinction between a trauma-related phenomena versus a complex cyclical affective disorder is perhaps moot.

Behavioral or Motoric Reenactments

Traumatic memories can be reenacted motorically, often with little or no awareness or insight into the nature of these behaviors. There is no specific medication to block these behaviors. However, they usually occur in the context of hyperarousal. Thus, they may be controlled by decreasing arousal and improving the patient's ability to modulate states of arousal. This is attempted in the manner discussed previously—with TCAs, MAOIs, clonazepam, clonidine, fluoxetine, and (in extreme cases) low-dose neuroleptics. If they occur in the context of marked impulsivity, then lithium or carbamazepine would be reasonable options. Also, if Saporta and van der Kolk are correct in speculating that these behaviors are released by malfunction of the brain's behavioral inhibition system caused by decreased serotonin function, then these behaviors should respond to serotonergic agonists (Saporta and van der Kolk, in press; van der Kolk and Saporta, in press). Unfortunately, there are no current empirical data that support or refute this prediction.

Dissociative Symptoms

There are no medications specific for dissociation. However, dissociative reactions usually occur in response to overwhelming arousal and affects. Thus, medications that improve the modulation of arousal and affects may reduce the patient's need to resort to dissociative mechanisms of defense. Antianxiety medications may reduce the "switching" process in patients with MPD when switching is driven by anxiety. Antianxiety medications such as clonazepam may be effective in treating patients with chronic depersonalization. Temporal lobe epilepsy should be ruled out in patients with dissociative symptoms (Benson et al. 1986; Mesulam 1981). We have not found carbamazepine effective in decreasing dissociative symptoms in patients who do not have epilepsy. The role of antipsychotic medications in dissociative disorders was discussed in a previous section. Loewenstein (1991) has published a more extensive discussion of psychopharmacology in the treatment of MPD.

Medications such as barbiturates or benzodiazepines are sometimes advocated for cases of psychogenic amnesia or fugue or to recover lost memories. Generally, amobarbital is used in the so-called "Amytal interview" and may be useful for diagnostic purposes (Perry and Jacobs 1982). We do not recommend such coerced recovery of memories other than in extreme circumstances. The patient may lack more healthy coping mechanisms for dealing with what is forgotten; forced retrieval with medications or hypnosis could lead to more pathological coping strategies (i.e., destructive acting out or psychosis). In general, we recommend working on coping strategies and a gradual, safe recovery of memories.

Self-Mutilation

Self-mutilating behaviors are highly indicative of a history of childhood trauma (Green 1978; Pattison and Kahan 1983). It has also been noted in traumatized adults without a history of child abuse (Greenspan and Samuel 1989; Pitman 1990). Because this behavior is associated with decreased serotonin function (Brown et al. 1979; Coccaro et al. 1989), fluoxetine and other serotonergic agonists should theoretically be effective. This has not been studied. Carbamazepine was shown to be effective for treatment of these behaviors in a study of BPD patients (Cowdry and Gardner 1988; Gardner and Cowdry 1986). Lithium may also help (Wickman and Reed 1987). We find lithium occasionally helpful, particularly when the behaviors are impulsive. Because this behavior is also frequently an attempt to decrease intense arousal, affect, or dissociation, it may help to improve modulation of affect and arousal with medications, as we described previously. We have found clonidine occasionally helpful for these behaviors in the context of high arousal. The endogenous opioid system is thought to be involved in these behaviors, and opiate receptor blockers have been found to decrease self-destructive behaviors in other populations (Herman et al. 1987). Unfortunately, not enough is known to recommend their routine use in the population considered here. Finally, low-dose neuroleptics may help where other regimens fail.

Sleep Disorders

Sleep disorders are extremely common in traumatized patients. Insomnia may be primarily due to the abnormal arousal of PTSD or may be due to nightmares, traumatic associations with the bedroom, or associations to time of night in which abuses occurred. Insomnia may also be secondary to other psychiatric syndromes, such as early morning awakening due to endogenous depression.

The approach to treatment of sleep disturbances in these patients is similar in certain respects to the approach to primary insomnia. Contributing medical conditions and drug side effects should be ruled out. The physician educates the patient regarding sleep hygiene and inventories the patient's use of stimulants such as caffeine and chocolate. Where bedtime is associated with traumatic events and thus triggers flashbacks and anxiety, psychological interventions that attempt to reframe bedtime routines may help. When insomnia is secondary to other psychiatric syndromes, treatment is directed to the primary psychopathology.

When insomnia is a primary PTSD symptom and where other interventions fail, pharmacologic intervention is called for. At times, managing other PTSD symptoms such as hyperarousal and flashbacks with various antidepressants, fluoxetine, clonazepam, and the like will resolve the sleep disturbance. However, insomnia or nightmares are often an isolated or persistent symptom requiring a specific focus. We find trazodone frequently effective in improving sleep and controlling nightmares, in doses from 25 to 100 mg at bedtime. This medication can be combined with other agents and may thus help to decrease insomnia that is exacerbated by medications such as fluoxetine. When trazodone fails or is not tolerated, benzodiazepines may be tried. We have had success with clonazepam and lorazepam in this regard. Hopefully, these pharmacologic interventions will be short-term. However, many patients have chronic sleep disturbances that require long-term treatment.

Medication Combinations

Medication combinations are frequently indicated in treating traumatized patients. This may occur when multiple target symptoms require treatment. For example, a patient's symptoms of depression and flashbacks may require a combination of fluoxetine and clonazepam; depression and impulsive self-mutilation may respond to fluoxetine plus lithium, and so on. Another reason for combination strategies would be to augment the effects of an agent, such as augmenting antidepressant response by adding lithium. Finally, medications may be combined to manage side effects. Examples include treating fluoxetine-induced insomnia with trazodone or treating akathisia with propranolol.

The physician must take care not to overmedicate the patient and to be alert to drug interactions. When complicated symptoms are resistant to medications, it may be difficult to decide whether to continue "chasing" these symptoms with multiple medications and thus risk the problems of "polypharmacy" or to restrain the use of medications and help the patient bear his or her discomfort by other means. This often occurs in the context of depression in the early phase of recovering traumatic memories. The decision as to how aggressively to pursue symptoms with medication combinations is a complex one and should involve an open discussion of the matter with the patient and his or her therapist.

Problems in Integrating Medications and Psychotherapy

Who Decides?

The patient, the therapist, and the medicating physician (when the physician is someone other than the therapist) should be active in decisions about whether or not to use medications. The decision should not be delegated solely to the pharmacologic consultant. The patient and the therapist may be in the best position to decide whether the patient's symptoms are sufficiently disruptive to his or her ability to use psychotherapy and sufficiently disruptive in daily life to warrant a trial of medication. The pharmacologist as consultant may advise them as to whether the symptoms in question are likely to be responsive to medication. The pharmacologist may also diagnose symptoms of coexisting psychiatric syndromes that require medical intervention. It is most important to engage the patient as an active participant in the decision to use medications, the determination of target symptoms, and the decision to discontinue medicines. In this way, we avoid a reenactment of the patient's past, where he or she passively endured something that was being done *to* him or her.

Addressing the Meaning of Medications in Therapy

Once medications are begun, issues regarding medication should not be split off from the therapy. Therapy should address the patient's feelings about medications. Medications may have multiple meanings for these patients. They may view referral to a pharmacologist either as a sign of rejection by the therapist or as an offer of healing and an opportunity to deepen the therapeutic work. They may view the need for medication as failure and as confirmation that they have lost their autonomy and that their bodies are once again out of their control. Alternatively, they could be helped to see medications as an opportunity to gain greater control, mastery, and autonomy. Patients may concretize medications as a symbol of illness and defect, resulting in avoidance of medications because of feelings of shame.

A patient's feelings about medication can contain transference meanings as well. For example, persistent complaints that medications are not helpful may allude to the fact that the patient is not finding the therapist helpful. It may suggest that the patient is unconsciously attempting to communicate to the therapist how helpless he or she feels by making the therapist feel equally helpless through projective identification. The opportunity to elaborate and explore these issues is missed if the therapist declines to discuss medication-related problems and refers these questions exclusively to the prescribing physician.

The ongoing need for medications should also be continually reassessed in therapy. Patients may cling to certain medications in an attempt to avoid all feeling. We do recognize, though, that some patients may need medications indefinitely.

The Meaning of Medications for the Therapist

Medications have meaning for therapists as well. Therapists should be aware of the potential for medications to carry countertransference feelings and actions. Pharmacologists should be aware of the role that medications can play in the therapeutic relationship in order to better assess a referral for psychopharmacology.

A therapist may think he or she has failed if a patient needs medications. If the therapist is unaware of these feelings, he or she is at risk of subtly acting out resentment. A referral for medications may also represent the therapist's difficulties in bearing the affects and memories emerging in the treatment. Medications may serve to titrate closeness or distance in the therapeutic relationship. A therapist may participate with the patient in reenacting abuse by pressuring him or her to take medications or, alternatively, by insisting that the patient endure symptoms without the aid of medications. This may occur when patient and therapist collude in a projective identification. Ideally, referral for medications is based on the therapist's realistic clinical assessment.

It is not unreasonable in certain circumstances for physicians treating trauma survivors in psychotherapy to have another psychiatrist manage the medications. This may be helpful with characterologically disturbed patients whose psychotherapy is complex and who are prone to intense and chaotic transference reactions. Some of these patients are prone to act in order not to feel, and their urgency to act can influence their therapists. This can lead prescribing therapists to add or change medications impulsively and inappropriately. Having a colleague manage the medications in these circumstances helps relieve the therapist's countertransference need to act and allows the therapist to model patience and the capacity to tolerate difficult feelings. However, other patients have such difficulty with trust that they will accept medications only from their therapists, often after much time and work spent on establishing a therapeutic alliance.

Finally, some patients may present for pharmacologic consultation who are in a flooded or intrusive stage of a posttraumatic syndrome because they are being pushed or are pushing themselves to remember too much, too fast. In these cases, the patient may not need medications if the therapeutic work can be redirected away from uncovering traumatic memories and toward a focus on coping, learning to bear feelings in the here and now, and recovering memories at a slower, safer pace.

Evaluating the Efficacy of Medications

In evaluating the efficacy of medications, therapists may ask themselves the following questions. Do the medications forward or hinder the process of therapy? Do the medications promote safer remembering and working-through, or do they promote maladaptive denial and avoidance? Is the patient more able to function in his or her daily life? Is the patient's sense of competence, control, and emotional well-being enhanced? Is he or she more able to engage in satisfying interpersonal relationships? Again, the patient must be actively involved in making these determinations.

Conclusion

In this chapter we have presented a model for the role of medications in treating adults who have been traumatized as children. We suggest that medications may decrease posttraumatic symptoms that impair the patient's capacity to utilize psychotherapy, and they may improve the patient's quality of life. According to current biological models for posttraumatic stress, we also suggest that medications restore the patient's capacity to modulate certain basic neurobiological functions that have been disrupted by overwhelming stress.

We have much to learn in this area. Although the medications we have reviewed may help many of these patients, there is a need for specific research focused on this population in order to devise more effective pharmacologic strategies. Finally, we have discussed various psychodynamic and interpersonal issues that may arise when integrating medications into the psychotherapy of trauma survivors. We hope that this discussion will help clinicians avoid injudicious use of medications and maximize the most effective integration of medications into psychotherapy when indicated.

References

Anisman HL, Ritch M, Sklar LS: Noradrenergic and dopaminergic interactions in escape behavior. Psychopharmacology (Berlin) 74:263–268, 1981

Anisman HL, Sklar LS: Catecholamine depletion in mice upon reexposure to stress: mediation of the escape deficits produced by inescapable shock. Journal of Comparative and Physiological Psychology 93:610–625, 1979

Asberg M, Traskman L, Thoren R: 5-HIAA in the cerebrospinal fluid: a biochemical suicide predictor. Arch Gen Psychiatry 33:93–97, 1976

Benson DF, Miller BL, Signer SF: Dual personality associated with epilepsy. Arch Neurol 43:471–474, 1986

Blanchard EB, Kolb LC, Pallemeyer BA, et al: A psychophysiologic study of post traumatic stress disorder in Vietnam veterans. Psychiatr Q 54:220–229, 1982

Breese GR, Cooper BR, Mueller RA: Evidence for involvement of 5-hydroxytryptamine in the actions of amphetamine. Br J Pharmacol 52:307–314, 1974

Brown GL, Goodwin FK, Ballenger JC, et al: Aggression in humans correlates with cerebrospinal fluid metabolites. Psychiatry Res 1:131–139, 1979

Brown GR, Anderson B: Psychiatric morbidity in adult inpatients with childhood histories of sexual and physical abuse. Am J Psychiatry 148:55–61, 1991

Cassens G, Roffman M, Kuruc A, et al: Alterations in brain norepinephrine metabolism induced by environmental stimuli previously paired with inescapable shock. Science 209:1138–1140, 1980

Charney DS, Menkes DB, Heninger GR. Receptor sensitivity and the mechanism of action of antidepressant treatment: implications for the etiology and therapy of depression. Arch Gen Psychiatry 38:1160–1180, 1981

Coccaro EF, Siever LJ, Klar HM, et al: Serotonergic studies in patients with affective and personality disorders: correlates with suicidal and impulsive aggressive behavior. Arch Gen Psychiatry 6:587–599, 1989

Coid J, Allolio B, Rees LH: Raised plasma metenkephalin in patients who habitually mutilate themselves. Lancet 2:545–546, 1983

Coons PM, Bowman ES, Pellow TA, et al: Posttraumatic aspects of the treatment of victims of sexual abuse and incest. Psychiatr Clin North Am 12:325–335, 1989

Coons PM, Cole C, Pellow TA, et al: Symptoms of posttraumatic stress and dissociation in women victims of abuse, in Incest-Related Syndromes of Adult Psychopathology. Edited by Kluft RP. Washington, DC, American Psychiatric Press, 1990, pp 55–74

Cornelius JR, Soloff PH, Perel JM, et al. Fluoxetine trial in borderline personality disorder. Psychopharmacol Bull 26:151–154, 1990

Cowdry RW, Gardner DL: Pharmacotherapy of borderline personality disorder: alprazolam, carbamazepine, trifluoperazine, and tranylcypromine. Arch Gen Psychiatry 45:111–119, 1988

Damlouji NF, Ferguson JM. Three cases of posttraumatic anorexia nervosa. Am J Psychiatry 142:362–363, 1985

Davidson J, Kudler H, Smith R, et al: Treatment of posttraumatic stress disorder with amitriptyline and placebo. Arch Gen Psychiatry 47:259–266, 1990

Davis M, Sheard MH: p-Chloroamphetamine (PCA): acute and chronic effects on habituation and sensitization of the acoustic startle response in rats. Eur J Pharmacol 135:261–273, 1976

Demitrack MA, Putnam FW, Brewerton TD, et al: Relation of clinical variables to dissociative phenomena in eating disorders. Am J Psychiatry 147:1184–1188, 1990

Depue RA, Spoont MR: Conceptualizing a serotonin trait: a behavioral dimension of constraint. Ann N Y Acad Sci 487:46–62, 1986

Dobbs D, Wilson WP. Observations on the persistence of traumatic war neurosis. Journal of Mental and Nervous Disorders 21:40–46, 1960

Enas GG, Pope HG, Levine LR: Fluoxetine in bulimia nervosa: double-blind study, in New Research Program and Abstracts of the American Psychiatric Association. Washington, DC, American Psychiatric Association, 1989

Famularo R, Kinscherff R, Fenton T: Propranolol treatment for childhood posttraumatic stress disorder; acute type. American Journal of Disorders of Childhood 142:1244–1247, 1988

Fanselow MS: Conditioned fear-induced opiate analgesia: a competing motivational state theory of stress analgesia. Ann N Y Acad Sci 467:40–54, 1986

Fesler FA: Valproate in combat-related posttraumatic stress disorder. J Clin Psychiatry 52:361–364, 1991

Frank JB, Kosten TR, Giller EL, et al: A randomized clinical trial of phenelzine and imipramine for posttraumatic stress disorder. Am J Psychiatry 145:1289–1291, 1988

Friedman MJ: Toward a rational pharmacotherapy of posttraumatic stress disorder: an interim report. Am J Psychiatry 145:281–285, 1988

Gardner DL, Cowdry RW: Positive effects of carbamazepine on behavioral dyscontrol in borderline personality disorder. Am J Psychiatry 143:519–522, 1986

Gardner DL, Cowdry RW: Pharmacotherapy of borderline personality disorder: a review. Psychopharmacol Bull 25:505–523, 1989

Gerson SC, Baldessarini RJ: Motor effects of serotonin in the central nervous system. Life Sci 27:1436–1451, 1980

Giral P, Martin P, Soubrié P, et al: Reversal of helpless behavior in rats by putative 5-HT1A agonists. Biol Psychiatry 23:237–242, 1988

Goldfarb LA: Sexual abuse antecedent to anorexia nervosa, bulimia, and compulsive overeating: three case reports. International Journal of Eating Disorders 6:675–680, 1987

Goodwin JM: Post-traumatic symptoms in incest victims, in Posttraumatic Stress Disorder in Children. Edited by Eth S, Pynoos RS. Washington, DC, American Psychiatric Press, 1985, pp 165–158

Gray JF: The Neuropsychology of Anxiety: An Enquiry Into the Functions of the Septo-hippocampal System. New York, Oxford University Press, 1987

Green AH: Self-destructive behavior in battered children. Am J Psychiatry 135:579–582, 1978

Greenspan GS, Samuel SE: Self-cutting after rape. Am J Psychiatry 146:789–790, 1989

Herman BH, Hammock MK, Arthur-Smith MA, et al: Naltrexone decreases self-injurious behavior. Ann Neurology 22:530–534, 1987

Herman J, van der Kolk BA: Traumatic antecedents of borderline personality, in Psychological Trauma. Edited by van der Kolk BA. Washington, DC, American Psychiatric Press, 1987, pp 111–126

Herman JL, Perry JC, van der Kolk BA: Childhood trauma in borderline personality disorder. Am J Psychiatry 46:490–495, 1989

Hodge GK, Butcher LL: 5-hydroxytryptamine correlates of isolation-induced aggression in mice. Eur J Pharmacol 28:236–237, 1974

Hogben GL, Cornfield RB: Treatment of traumatic war neurosis with phenelzine. Arch Gen Psychiatry 38:440–445, 1981

Horowitz MJ: Stress Response Syndromes, 2nd Edition. Northvale, NJ, Jason Aronson, 1986

Keane TM, Albano AM, Blake DD: Current trends in the treatment of posttraumatic stress symptoms, in Torture and Its Consequences: Current Treatment Approaches. Edited by Basoglu M. Cambridge, England, Cambridge University Press (in press)

Kluft RP: First rank symptoms as a diagnostic clue to multiple personality disorder. Am J Psychiatry 144:293–298, 1987

Kolb L: Neuropsychological hypothesis explaining posttraumatic stress disorder. Am J Psychiatry 144:989–995, 1987

Kolb LC, Burris B, Griffiths S: Propranolol and clonidine in treatment of the chronic posttraumatic stress of war, in Posttraumatic Stress Disorder: Psychological and Biological Sequela. Edited by van der Kolk BA. Washington DC, American Psychiatric Press, 1984

Kosten TR, Krystal J: Biological mechanisms in posttraumatic stress disorder: relevance to substance abuse, in Recent Developments in Alcoholism. Edited by Galanter M. New York, Plenum, 1988

Kosten TR, Mason JW, Giller RB, et al: Sustained urinary norepinephrine and epinephrine elevation in posttraumatic stress disorder. Psychoneuroendocrinology 12:13–20, 1987

Kraemer GW, Ebert MH, Lake CR, et al: Hypersensitivity to d-amphetamine several years after early social deprivation in rhesus monkeys. Psychopharmacology (Berlin) 82:266–271, 1984

Krystal JH, Kosten TR, Perry BD, et al: Neurobiological aspects of PTSD: review of clinical and preclinical studies. Behavior Therapy 20:177–198, 1989

Lerer B, Bleich A, Kotler M, et al: Posttraumatic stress disorder in Israeli combat veterans: effect of phenelzine treatment. Arch Gen Psychiatry 44:976–981, 1987a

Lerer B, Ebstein RP, Shestasky M, et al: Cyclic AMP signal transduction in posttraumatic stress disorder. Am J Psychiatry 144:1324–1327, 1987b

Lewis JW, Cannon JT, Liebeskind JC: Opioid and opioid mechanisms of stress analgesia. Science 208:623–625, 1980

Liebowitz MR, Quitkin FM, Stewart JW, et al: Antidepressant specificity in atypical depression. Arch Gen Psychiatry 45:129–137, 1988

Links PS, Steiner M, Boiago I, et al: Lithium therapy for borderline patients: preliminary findings. Journal of Personality Disorders 4:173–181, 1990

Lipper S, Davidson JR, Grady TA, et al: Preliminary study of carbamazepine in posttraumatic stress disorder. Psychosomatics 26:849–854, 1986

Loewenstein RJ: Rational psychopharmacology in the treatment of multiple personality disorder. Psychiatr Clin North Am 14:721–740, 1991

Loewenstein RJ, Hornstein N, Farber B: Open trial of clonazepam in the treatment of PTSD symptoms in multiple personality disorder. Dissociation 1:3–12, 1988

Maier SF: Stressor control and stress-induced analgesia. Ann N Y Acad Sci 467:55–72, 1986

Maier SF, Seligman ME: Learned helplessness: theory and evidence. J Exp Psychology [Gen] 105:3–46, 1976

McFall ME, Murburg M, Grant NK, et al: Autonomic responses to stress in veterans with posttraumatic stress disorder. Biol Psychiatry 27:1165–1175, 1990

Mesulam M: Dissociative states with abnormal temporal lobe EEG—multiple personality and the illusion of possession. Arch Neurol 38:176–181, 1981

Norden MJ: Fluoxetine in borderline personality disorder. Prog Neuropsychopharmacol Biol Psychiatry 13:885–893, 1989

Ogata SN, Silk KR, Goodrich S, et al: Childhood sexual and physical abuse in adult patients with borderline personality disorder. Am J Psychiatry 147:1008–1013, 1990

Paige SR, Reid GM, Allen MG, et al: Psychophysiologic correlates of posttraumatic stress disorder. Biol Psychiatry 27:419–430, 1990

Pattison EM, Kahan J: The deliberate self-harm syndrome. Am J Psychiatry 140:867–872, 1983

Perry BD, Giller EL, Southwick SM: Altered plasma alpha-2-adrenergic receptor affinity states in PTSD. Am J Psychiatry 144:1511–1512, 1987

Perry JC, Jacobs D: Overview: clinical applications of the Amytal interview in psychiatric emergency settings. Am J Psychiatry 139:552–559, 1982

Pitman RK: Self-mutilation in combat-related PTSD (letter). Am J Psychiatry 147:123–134, 1990

Pitman RK, Orr S, Forque DF, de Jong JB, et al: Psychophysiologic assessment of posttraumatic stress disorder imagery in Vietnam combat veterans. Arch Gen Psychiatry 144:970–975, 1987

Pitman RK, Orr S, Forgue D, et al: Psychophysiologic responses to combat imagery of Vietnam veterans with posttraumatic stress disorder versus other anxiety disorders. J Abnorm Psychol 99:49–54, 1990a

Pitman RK, van der Kolk BA, Orr SP, et al. Naloxone-reversible analgesic response to combat-related stimuli in posttraumatic stress disorder: a pilot study. Arch Gen Psychiatry 47:541–547, 1990b

Poschlova N, Masek K, Krsiak M. Amphetamine-like effects of 5,6-dihydroxytryptamine in social behavior in the mouse. Neuropharmacology 16:317–321, 1977

Post RM, Kopanda RT: Cocaine, kindling, and psychosis. Am J Psychiatry 133:627–634, 1976

Putnam FW: Diagnosis and Treatment of Multiple Personality Disorder. New York, Guilford, 1989

Quitkin FM, McGrath PJ, Stewart JW, et al: Phenelzine and imipramine in mood reactive depressives: further delineation of the syndrome of atypical depression. Arch Gen Psychiatry 46:787–793, 1989

Rainey JM, Aleem A, Ortiz A, et al: Laboratory procedures for the inducement of flashbacks. Am J Psychiatry 144:1317–1319, 1987

Reist C, Kauffman CD, Haier RJ, et al: A controlled trial of desipramine in 18 men with posttraumatic stress disorder. Am J Psychiatry 146:513–516, 1989

Rifkin A, Quitkin F, Carrillo C, et al: Lithium carbonate in emotionally unstable character disorder. Arch Gen Psychiatry 27:519–523, 1972

Samanin R, Garattini S: The serotonergic system in the brain and its possible functional connections with other aminergic systems. Life Sci 17:1201–1210, 1976

Saporta JA, Jr, van der Kolk BA: Psychobiological consequences of severe trauma, in Torture and Its Consequences: Current Treatment Approaches. Edited by Basoglu M. Cambridge, England, Cambridge University Press (in press)

Schetky DH: A review of the literature on the long-term effects of sexual abuse, in Incest-Related Syndromes of Adult Psychopathology. Edited by Kluft RP. Washington, DC, American Psychiatric Press, 1990, pp 35–54

Sheard MH: Effect of lithium on human aggression. Nature 230:113–114, 1971

Sherman AD, Petty F: Neurochemical basis of the action of antidepressants on learned helplessness. Behav Neural Biol 30:119–134, 1980

Shestatsky M, Greenberg D, Lerer B: A controlled trial of phenelzine in posttraumatic stress disorder. Psychiatry Res 24:149–155, 1988

Soloff PH: Psychopharmacologic therapies in borderline personality disorders, in American Psychiatric Press Review of Psychiatry, Vol 8. Edited by Tasman A, Hales RE, Francis AJ. Washington, DC, American Psychiatric Press, 1989

Soubrié P: Reconciling the role of central serotonin neurons in human and animal behavior. Behavioral and Brain Sciences 9:319–364, 1986

Southwick SM, Yehuda R, Giller EL, et al: Altered platelet alpha-2-adrenergic receptor binding sites in borderline personality disorder. Am J Psychiatry 147:1014–1017, 1990

Southwick SM, Yehuda R, Giller EL: Characterization of depression in war-related posttraumatic stress disorder. Am J Psychiatry 148:179–183, 1991

Valzelli L: Aggressive behavior induced by isolation, in Aggressive Behavior. Edited by Garattini S, Sigg L. Amsterdam, Exerpta Medica, 1969

Valzelli L: Serotonergic inhibitory control of experimental aggression. Psychopharmacological Research Communications 14:1–13, 1982

Valzelli L, Bernasconi S: Aggressiveness by isolation and brain serotonin turnover changes in different strains of mice. Neuropsychobiology 5:129–135, 1979 van Kammen DP: 5-HT: a neurotransmitter for all seasons? Biol Psychiatry 22:1–3, 1987

van der Kolk BA: Psychopharmacological issues in post-traumatic stress disorder. Hosp Community Psychiatry 34:683–691, 1983

van der Kolk BA: The drug treatment of posttraumatic stress disorder. J Affective Disord 13:203–213, 1987

van der Kolk BA: The compulsion to repeat the trauma: reenactment, revictimization, and masochism. Psychiatr Clin North Am 12:389–411, 1989

van der Kolk BA, Saporta JA: The biological response to psychic trauma, in Handbook on Posttraumatic Stress. Edited by Rafael, B. New York, Plenum (in press)

van der Kolk BA, Greenberg MS, Boyd H, et al: Inescapable shock, neurotransmitters, and addiction to trauma: toward a psychobiology of posttraumatic stress. Biol Psychiatry 20:314–325, 1985

van der Kolk BA, Greenberg MS, Orr SP, et al: Endogenous opioids, stress-induced analgesia, and posttraumatic stress disorder. Psychopharmacol Bull 25:417–421, 1989

Walsh BT, Hadigan CM, Devlin MJ, et al: Long-term outcome of antidepressant treatment for bulimia nervosa. Am J Psychiatry 148:1206–1212, 1991

Weiss JM, Glazer HI, Pohorecky LA, et al: Effects of chronic exposure to stressors on subsequent avoidance-escape behavior and on brain norepinephrine. Psychosom Med 37:522–524, 1975

Welch AS, Welch BL: Isolation, reactivity, and aggression: evidence for an involvement of brain catecholamines and serotonin, in Physiology of Aggression and Defeat. Edited by Eleftheriou BE, Scott JP. New York, Plenum, 1971

Wickman EA, Reed JV: Lithium for the control of aggressive and self-mutilating behavior. Int Clin Psychopharmacol 2:181–190, 1987

Winslow JT, Insel TR: Neurobiology of obsessive compulsive disorder: a possible role for serotonin. J Clin Psychiatry 51(suppl):27–35, 1990

Wolf ME, Alavi A, Mosnaim AD: Posttraumatic stress disorder in Vietnam veterans clinical and EEG findings: possible therapeutic effects of carbamazepine. Biol Psychiatry 23:642–644, 1988

Chapter 6

The Seduction Hypothesis 100 Years After

Jean M. Goodwin, M.D., M.P.H.

*A*s we approach the centennial of the Seduction Hypothesis, it is gratifying at last to have data about treatment and treatment outcomes in patients who were sexually victimized in childhood. The preliminary debate about whether such survivors of sexual abuse existed has lasted so long. We are almost a century late in answering Freud's original 1896 question about whether specific treatment focused on the childhood abuse could resolve the numerous and severe symptoms found in these individuals.

In fact, much of what has been written in the past 97 years has remained within the phenomenological confines of Freud's original and brilliant observations, saved from oblivion (somewhat to the chagrin of everyone involved, feminists and psychoanalysts alike) by the women's movement of the 1960s and 1970s.

In 1896, Freud knew that, in his 18 patients who described childhood seductions, symptoms were various and multiple (Masson 1984). He described anxiety attacks, genital pain and paresthesias, premature and aggressive sexuality, problems with defecation and eating (he thought the eating problems were related to forced fellatio), hysterical conversion symptoms, obsessive self-reproach, and paranoia. Each symptom had the property of fitting into the narrative of the abuse like a piece in a jigsaw puzzle. Some detail of the symptom's timing, sequencing, affective tone, or sensation would precisely recapitulate some lost detail of the childhood abuse.

Freud predicted that the severity of the symptoms would vary with the severity of the abuse (particularly with total number of incidents) and that children abused before age 8 were at special risk for symptom formation. He thought that symptoms represented a summation of the traumatic force of the experience, the presence of a hypnoid state in the child (based on his colleague Breuer's thinking, which in turn was influenced by Janet), the child's associations to the experience, and constitutional factors. Not every child who was sexually abused would experience symptoms. Triggers, especially the sexual behaviors encountered in courtship, might initiate or exacerbate symptoms.

Freud proposed that every case of hysteria resulted from childhood sexual abuse. There were problems with this Koch's postulate approach to the data. Freud was already seeing problems other than hysteria in his patients—obsessions, paranoia, no visible symptoms at all. So, not everyone with trauma would develop "hysteria." On the other hand, "hysteria" was such a vague, inclusive category at that time that even Freud would have had to concede that not everyone diagnosed as having hysteria would have experienced trauma. The theorizing was rigid and unworkable, but it must be remembered that the biopsychosocial model had not yet been invented.

Others raised credibility problems. Freud initially discounted these objections, pointing out that the sexual abuse accounts he heard felt credible to him because of the patients' reluctance and shame about disclosure, their violent reexperiencing of emotions and sensation at times when disclosing, their tendency to derealize and redissociate after disclosing, the detail in the disclosures, and the contextualization of the sexual disclosure within the rest of the childhood history, including childhood symptoms and relationships.

Freud had found it convincing, too, when witnesses or abusers came in to confirm the patient's account in two of his cases. In answer to the question of whether he himself was implanting these sexual stories in the patients' minds, Freud said he never succeeded in finding what he expected; maybe others knew how to do that, but he did not.

Much of incest research in the past 20 years has entailed putting percentages and P values on these original observations. We now know (in more statistical detail than did Freud) that survivors of childhood sexual abuse are at greater risk for anxiety disorders, sexual dysfunction, eating disorders, unexplained somatic symptoms, and low self-esteem (Briere 1989; Goodwin 1989, 1990, 1993; Goodwin and Attias, in press). We know that the severe dissociative symptoms seem to cluster in those victimized before age 8 (Kluft 1985). We know that severity of trauma correlates with severity of symptoms (Herman et al. 1986);

that some survivors are asymptomatic; and that in more than two-thirds of cases, confirmatory data (witnesses, confessions, material evidence) can be found if sought (Herman and Schatzow 1987). There remains enough yet unexplored in Freud's paper to occupy phenomenologists for another generation.

What about treatment? Treatment failure was the linchpin in Freud's own subsequent arguments against his original theory (Masson 1984). Freud's patients were not able to terminate their analyses successfully. They fled treatment. Their symptoms persisted. Freud had other cogent problems with his theory. His clinical experience did not fit with the known epidemiology of incest, which was supposed to be vanishingly rare. It took us 80 years to repair those epidemiologic errors (Russell 1986). Freud had clinical problems when reconstructing sexual scenes because of the difficulty in differentiating occurrences from fantasies. A closer reading of Janet would have helped him here. Janet saw clearly that one must reconstruct not only the fragmented traumatic event but also the fragmented rescue fantasies, revenge fantasies, escape fantasies, symptomatic symbolizations, and day and night dreams about the event. We are putting together several jigsaw puzzles simultaneously, not just one. Freud also had a problem with his theory of memory. He believed he was helping patients retrieve intact memories that had been pushed away, behind what he conceptualized as a repression barrier. We now know that some of the memories are fragmented from the beginning and must be reconstructed quite literally in order to be experienced and then remembered.

These other problems were real, but it was the treatment failures that most troubled Freud. When Ferenczi began treating such patients 35 years later, Freud was shocked at the treatment modifications that Ferenczi introduced in order to achieve better therapeutic success (Masson 1984). Ferenczi probably was dealing with a more severely abused group than Freud had encountered. Substance abuse, ego-splitting, and identification with the aggressor were more prominent in this group. Some had been abused sadistically, starting in infancy. Split-off child alters would appear in sessions screaming for help or reexperiencing Ferenczi as the abuser. Ferenczi responded by treating these fragments as if they were real children, letting them sit on his lap and hug and kiss him. Freud said that such boundary violations would prove disastrous for the analyst, for psychoanalysis in general, and ultimately for the patient.

What this book tells us is that both Freud and Ferenczi were right in a way: Treatment does take a long time, and it does have to be modified—though not in the way Ferenczi thought. Necessary modifications include the following:

1. Acknowledgement of the centrality in the treatment of the benevolent relationship with the therapist;
2. Attention to the extreme psychophysiological pain of the patient;
3. Openness to the use of child therapy techniques, particularly play and expressive therapies and use of collateral data sources and a multimodal treatment plan; and
4. Awareness of the hypnoid state changes present in some patients, and attention to helping the patient respond to these adaptively.

In Chapter 1, Gelinas provides a persuasive picture of the power of that benevolent therapeutic relationship, which may be the abuse survivor's first experience of being listened to, understood, valued, encouraged, and helped. This goes far beyond what is at times referred to dismissively as being "supportive." Its theoretical base reaches back to Fairbairn and Winnicott; the therapist becomes a "good object" and survives the patient's attempts (and the introjected abuser's attempts) to destroy this new possibility for goodness and creativity. Kohut's ideas are also helpful; these patients have not been mirrored and have not been able to share their ambitions or ideals. Trust must be earned and sometimes created in the treatment. The survivor is in no position to bestow it except in the form of split-off, conditional, temporary, false-self compliance.

Such patients often do leave treatment, because their emotional pain is severe. Some symptoms of terrorization (e.g., the posttraumatic symptoms described in Chapter 2) may be untouched even by good treatment that is effective against other symptom complexes. Treatment may act as a trigger and intensify symptoms. My experience is that effective treatment always involves a reenactment of some aspect of the abuse. The patient feels momentarily seduced or overcompliant or sexually stimulated in a treatment session. The better the therapy, the more quickly this can be noticed, interrupted, commented upon, explored, and connected to lost elements of the original traumatic situation or to persistent repeating patterns of pain or dysfunction. However, in real life, the process is awkward, ill-timed, and imperfect. Therapist and patient must learn to monitor basic functions, somatic sensations, and idiosyncratic manifestations of anxiety. All survivors need a crisis plan and a medical care plan. Having a hospitalization plan as a backup can help ensure that this will not be needed. Medication can be helpful here in taking enough of the edge off the pain to allow treatment to continue. It is in dealing with this intense posttraumatic intrapsychic pain that clinicians have been most hampered by the diagnostic confusion between these patients and patients with borderline personality disorder. These traumatized patients usually need more treatment when they ask for more treatment; they are being realistic, not manipulative.

Therapists who are skilled and comfortable working with children will do well with patients who were survivors of childhood sexual abuse. Because memories are interrupted and defective, they often do not yet exist in verbal form. Secrecy threats may have banned verbal expression specifically. Symbolic expression in drawings, sand play, or work in the patient's own creative medium may become possible before verbalization. When amnesia is a problem in present living as well as in reconstructing childhood memories, the therapist must have access to collateral forms of data. Those familiar with child work will easily grasp the resulting network of collaborators that may include family members; medical caregivers; providers of group, marital, or family therapy; pastors; crisis hotlines; friends; coaches; teachers; or co-workers. The therapist's evolving role as case manager allows modeling, coaching, and practicing of integrated functioning in a benevolent context (Turkus 1991).

It is in the more dissociated survivors that state change requires recognition and treatment. In our society, we like to pretend that our everyday, pragmatic executive state is not only our official persona but also the only one that exists. This is probably not true for anyone. Older cultures provide ritualized space and time for state changes to childlike regressions, grief states, ecstasies, or displays of anger and revenge (Ross 1991). Certainly, with survivors of childhood sexual abuse, it is not safe to assume a unitary identity, worldview, mood state, or philosophical stance. When the patient shifts into a parentified state, a therapist may feel manipulated. When the helpless child state supervenes, a therapist may feel abandoned without an active patient ally. A shift to the angry cynical state may leave the therapist feeling hopeless. When states are shifting rapidly, therapeutic work may become impossible, and the patient may become dangerously disoriented. Recognition and education about such state changes are critical for the treatment alliance.

If this is the agenda, how long does it take? Freud was trying to treat patients in 100 sessions or less. In many cases, this was not enough time. More important than quantity of hours is understanding what stage a particular patient is traversing. In Chapter 2, Paddison and colleagues describe three key phases or issues in therapy:

1. Symptom control or safety;
2. Narrative reconstruction of the traumatic childhood; and
3. Learning to live outside the world of abuse as it has persisted into adulthood or been recreated in relationships or symptomatology (Herman 1990; Putnam 1989).

Although treatment proceeds roughly from stage one to stage three, one is to some extent always working on all three phases simultaneously. For example, some limited trauma reconstruction may be necessary to understand life-threatening substance use or an eating disorder well enough to control it. However, it would be folly to plunge into full-time reconstructive work when basic functions like eating and sleeping are jeopardized; when reconstruction triggers symptoms, the focus on symptom control returns to center stage.

Much of the art of using the modalities described here involves careful timing. Recognition of dissociative state changes and judicious use of medication may be crucial initially in bringing a patient's symptoms under control. Participation in an incest group can be an important adjunct when narrating is the core task. In Chapter 1, Gelinas argues that some form of confrontation with the abuser, if only in fantasy, is a powerful way to complete the work of narration in a way that leads to changes in the skewed patterns of relating that have developed in the abusive environment. At this point, relearning becomes the central task. In this phase, Gelinas might encourage the patient to adopt a plant and experiment with the practice of benevolence toward this living thing, all the while differentiating the components of benevolence from the malevolent context in which the patient had to grow. In this phase, marital and sex therapy can be entered into with long-term goals in view, not merely crisis intervention.

Survivors will have their own endpoints for treatment. When there is a question about simplifying or discontinuing the treatment plan, it is clarifying to review progress in each of these three areas.

Successful termination includes anticipation of the possibility of future treatment needs. Continued normal development may produce new triggers that the survivor may need help to master. The Freudian case in which incest and malevolence are best documented was the one called "Wolf-Man." This young Russian aristocrat gave a history of generations of suicides, alcoholism, and abuse in his family. Although he benefited from treatment, his ongoing exposure to societal violence—the Russian Revolution, two World Wars, the Holocaust—produced retraumatization. His needs for treatment were lifelong (Goodwin et al. 1990).

As our data about natural history becomes statistical as well as anecdotal, we will understand more about the needs for lifelong intervention. Self-help groups, journal writing, self-analysis, exercise, and meditation techniques may be practicable at this level of tertiary prevention, as well as creating expressive art, participating actively in one's community, cultivating living things, experiencing the wilderness, contributing to philosophical traditions of meaning, and all the other activities that constitute the benevolent context that survivors are learning to inhabit.

References

Briere J: Therapy for Adults Molested as Children. New York, Springer, 1989

Goodwin J: Sexual Abuse: Incest Victims and Their Families. Chicago, IL, Mosby-Yearbook, 1989

Goodwin J: Applying to adult incest victims what we have learned from victimized children, in Incest-Related Syndromes of Adult Psychopathology. Edited by Kluft R. Washington, DC, American Psychiatric Press, 1990, pp 55–74

Goodwin J: Rediscovering Childhood Trauma: Historical Casebook and Clinical Applications. Washington, DC, American Psychiatric Press, 1993

Goodwin J, Attias R: Eating disorders in victims of multimodal child abuse, in Clinical Perspectives on Multiple Personality Disorder. Edited by Kluft R, Fine C. Washington, DC, American Psychiatric Press (in press)

Goodwin J, Hill S, Attias R: Historical and folkloric techniques of exorcism: applications to the treatment of dissociative disorders. Dissociation 3:214–217, 1990

Herman J: Discussion, in Incest-Related Syndromes of Adult Psychopathology. Edited by Kluft R. Washington, DC, American Psychiatric Press, 1990, pp 288–293

Herman J, Schatzow E: Recovery and verification of memories of childhood trauma. Psychoanalytic Psychology 4:1–14; 1987

Herman J, Russell D, Trocki K: Long-term effects of incestuous abuse in childhood. Am J Psychiatry 143:1293–1296, 1986

Kluft R: Childhood Antecedents of Multiple Personality. Washington, DC, American Psychiatric Press, 1985

Masson J: The Assault on Truth. New York, Farrar, Strauss & Giroux, 1984

Putnam F: Diagnosis and Treatment of Multiple Personality Disorder. New York, Guilford, 1989

Ross C: The dissociated executive self and the cultural dissociation barrier. Dissociation 4:55–61, 1991

Russell D: The Secret Trauma: Incest in the Lives of Girls and Women. New York, Basic Books, 1986

Turkus J: Psychotherapy and case management for multiple personality disorder: synthesis for continuity of care. Psychiatr Clin North Am 14:649–660, 1991

Index